INVISIBLE GUESTS

INVISIBLE GUESTS
The Development of Imaginal Dialogues

MARY WATKINS

WITH A PREFACE BY
ROBERT ROMANYSHYN

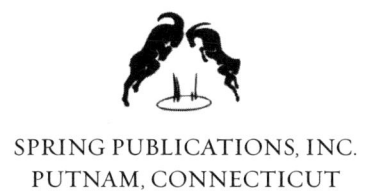

SPRING PUBLICATIONS, INC.
PUTNAM, CONNECTICUT

Copyright © 2000 by Mary Watkins
All rights reserved.

Published by Spring Publications, Inc.
28 Front Street, Suite 3
Putnam, CT 06260
www.springpublications.com

Originally published by the Analytic Press, Hillsdale, NJ, 1986
and subsequently by Sigo Press, Boston, 1990.

Third edition, second printing 2005

Printed in Canada
Cover design by white.room productions, New York

Cover image:
Wooden god from the Austral Islands, representing A'a, the principal deity of Rurutu. Inside the detachable back is a cavity where smaller images may be kept. Photograph by David Finn, from *Henry Moore at the British Museum*. New York: Harry N. Abrams, 1982 (reproduced with permission of the photographer).

ISBN-13: 978-0-88214-380-4
ISBN-10: 0-88214-380-8

Library of Congress Cataloging-in-Publication Data

Watkins, Mary M.
    Invisible guests : the development of imaginal dialogues / Mary Watkins.—[3rd ed.]
      p.   cm.
    Includes bibliographical references.
    ISBN-13: 978-0-88214-358-3 (pbk. : alk. paper)
    ISBN-10: 0-88214-358-1 (pbk. : alk. paper)
    1. Imaginary conversations—Psychological aspects. 2. Self-talk.   I. Title
BF697.5.S47 W37 2000
153.3'2—dc21   00-029157

∞ The paper used in this publication meets the minimum requirements of the American National Standard for Information Sciences—Permanence of Paper for Printed Library Materials, ANSI Z39.48-1992.

To

Bernard Kaplan
mentor, friend

CONTENTS

Preface .... *i*
Introduction 1

PART I

Themes in Contemporary Psychological Approaches to the Functions and Development of Imaginal Dialogues

1 Imaginal Dialogues and Reason 11
2 Reality and the Imagination 21
3 Seeing Imaginal Dialogues as Primitive 37

PART II

A Critique of Contemporary Psychological Approaches to Imaginal Dialogues

4 Imaginal Dialogues and Reason 49
5 Imagination as Reality 59
6 The Impact of Conceptions of Development on Approaching Imaginal Dialogues 81

PART III

Re-Conceiving a Developmental Theory of Imaginal Dialogues

7	"The Characters Speak Because They Want to Speak:" The Autonomy of the Imaginal Other	93
8	The Dialogues Between Multiple Characters; The Monologues of Multiple Personality	107
9	Character Development: The Articulation of the Imaginal Other	113
10	Relativizing the Ego and the Birth of Dialogue	121

PART IV

Therapeutic Implications: Entertaining Voices

11	The Voices of Hallucination	135
12	The Fish-Lady and the Little Girl: Case History Told From the Points of View of the Characters	155

Epilogue 177
Afterword 179
References 191

ACKNOWLEDGMENTS

My warmest thanks to friends and colleagues who took the time to read some or all of this text, to share with me their thoughts, criticisms, and encouragement: Bernard Kaplan, Leonard Cirillo, Seymour Wapner; Patricia Berry, Stuart Cane, Edward Casey, Joseph de Rivera, Lawrence Erlbaum, Mary Helen Sullivan, James Hillman, Gail Hornstein, Joan Klagsbrun, Eleanor Starke Kobrin, Lyndy Pye, Charles Scott, Randolph Severson, Angelyn Spignesi, Paul Stepansky, and Stanley Sultan. I am grateful to Robert Romanyshyn for writing the preface to this new editon.

My debts to fellow writers—so numerous—are noted in my text, though such references do not begin to display adequate gratitude for the companionship and conversation the reading of such works provide as one is trying to understand. Particularly helpful in orienting the arguments here were works by Bernard Kaplan, Henry Corbin, James Hillman, Edward Casey, Theodore Sarbin, M. H. Abrams, Martin Buber, Erving Goffman, and Erwin Straus.

And when the books and pen were put aside each day, Robert Rosenthal was always ready to add his wisdom to help me think through a point, to listen tirelessly to portions of the text that worried me, and to entertain invisible guests at our table. With such a home, writing can be a happiness.

PREFACE

Readers of the first edition of Mary Watkins' book, which appeared fourteen years ago, will undoubtedly recall the evocative and persuasive ways she demonstrated the autonomy of the imaginal other and the singular importance of dialogue in relation to invisible guests. Reading her book for a second time deepens those original impressions. But I would add here that this third edition offers more than another reading. It is a new book when one reads the text from the perspective of Watkins' Afterword. In my Preface, therefore, I want to encourage her readers to begin with the Afterword, to read it carefully, and then enter the text from its perspective.

What I find most provocative in this new edition is the expansion of imaginal dialogues to embrace not only our relations with others, but also our relations with the "beings of nature and the earth, and that which we take to be divine." Mary Watkins is quite correct to situate our dialogical relations with imaginal others as a "subtext of 'holy converse.'" This bold move opens the imaginal field to broader horizons and emphasizes how our encounters with the autonomous psyche always have something of a numinous or sacred quality to them. As the poet Rainer Maria Rilke reminds us, language is a vocation. We are called into speech by the other, a calling which presumes that one has first heard the other because one is listening. Holy converse as a subtext of imaginal dialogue is grounded in the receptive ear, in a posture which in lending an ear to the other is capable of being addressed, witnessed, embraced, and also challenged by the other.

Dialogue as openness to the other is a radically ethical way of being and living in the world. It is no surprise, therefore, that in the

Afterword Watkins sites the work of Paulo Freire. This Brazilian-born pedagogist has consistently shown us how true education must be a liberation of consciousness from its oppression by systems of speaking and thinking, operating as monologues that enforce obedient silence. In Freire's work we learn that the ethics of dialogue requires more than the multiplication of voices in the conversation. Such multiplication results only in an overload of information. Beyond it, what is required is that the one who speaks recognizes and acknowledges the contexts, with their unarticulated assumptions and values, of his or her words and thoughts. The presence of the other is always an occasion for this act of critical self-regard. In Freire's terms, the other, whether it be a dream figure or the homeless person on the street, or the caged animal is always the possibility of rupture, that moment of breakdown when critical self-regard can become a breakthrough for the appeal of the other to be heard.

In the Coda to the Afterword, Watkins writes that, "In the end, the direction of this book is not inward...only." This is the expansion I mentioned earlier, and it is this move out of psychological inwardness into an eco-cosmological relatedness which prompts me to call this third edition a new work. Depth psychology, particularly in its Jungian orientation, has always honored the autonomy of the psyche, but it too often imprisoned itself within the narrow confines of a psyche cut off from the other and the world. Watkins' phenomenological orientation moves depth psychology into that place where the other as difference is the depth of Self. The unconscious is between us and the notion of depth is radically relational and dialogical. We need this type of depth psychology today if we are to be ethically responsible human beings and ecologically responsive to those other and different voices of creation. The third edition of Watkins' book takes a bold step in that direction. Moreover, it traces between the first and third edition that beautiful arc which bears testimony to a mind, a heart, and a spirit which has faithfully followed its call. This is a book we need to read. But it is also one of those books where the need is also a pleasure.

—Robert D. Romanyshyn

INTRODUCTION

The purpose of poetry is to remind us
how difficult it is to remain just one person,
for our house is open, there are no keys to the doors,
and invisible guests come in and out at will.
—Czeslaw Milosz from "Ars Poetica"

In the Hebraic tradition human beings were distinguished from all other living creatures not by virtue of their capacity for reason but by virtue of their engagement in three kinds of dialogues: dialogues with neighbors, with themselves, and with God (Niebuhr, 1955). At first glance in our own time and culture, dialogues with ourselves and with the gods seem dim and almost silent next to our dialogues with our neighbors. These dialogues seem to flee from listening ears, hiding out in the most private parts of our solitude and fantasy. They abandon speaking aloud, or otherwise manifesting themselves, as though shrinking from the pejorative labels "pathological," "immature," or "superstitious." But if we approach without such critical predilections, we can begin again to hear the voices of these other dialogues—these, let us say, "imaginal dialogues."

Side by side and woven through our dialogues with our neighbors, these imaginal dialogues persist. We may find ourselves speaking with our reflection in the mirror, with the photograph of someone we miss, with a figure from a dream or a movie, with our dog. And even when we are outwardly silent, within the ebb and flux of our thought, we talk with critics, with our mothers, our god(s), our consciences; indeed we do so just as steadily as we once spoke to our dolls, our imaginary companions, the people of our painted pictures. We may find ourselves as audience or as narrator to conversations among imaginal others—others not physically present but actually experienced nonetheless. At times we may even notice ourselves playing more than one role in these imaginal dialogues—now child, now old one, abandoned one. These imaginal dialogues, their functions and lines of development, are the theme of this book.

Experientially imaginal dialogues can take several forms: conversation between a self and an imaginal other(s), between aspects of the Self such as "me" and "I," or between imaginal others with a self as audience to the imaginal scene. One might argue that these are not distinct classes of dialogue, that the category "conversation between aspects of the Self" logically subsumes the other two categories of "conversation between a self and an imaginal other" and "conversation between imaginal others." However, here they are treated separately so that we can begin to consider how the dramatic dialogues of thought are experienced, not just how they are conceived.

At times we argue with a critical part of ourselves; that is to say the critical voice sounds like us and is indistinguishable from that point of view we take to be our own. At other times we argue with a critic whose voice is that of a specific teacher—one known to us from daily life or perhaps from dream life, whose point of view is experienced as different from our usual one. To preserve these experiential distinctions, we shall define "Self" as the collection of different characters (or "self- and object-representations") who can be said to populate an individual's thoughts, feelings, and actions. In other words, the Self is that world of characters whom one entertains and/or identifies with. The "self" shall be used to designate that part of the Self one is identified with at a given moment. Hence, when it is said that a dialogue is being carried out between self and imaginal other, the self here is the experiential locus of consciousness associated with the feeling of "I." Its identity may shift, e.g., from counterdependent adult to whiny, wanting child. Insofar as some of these identifications are relatively stable over time, the term "habitual ego" shall be used. For instance a woman may have a habitual ego identification with a character (or self representation) who is strong, energetic, and willful.

In psychoanalytic parlance these imaginal others who are felt as presences and as ego/alien are called "introjects," while those who are closer to our self-representations are labeled "identifications." However, Meissner (1981) points out that these clear distinctions do not always parallel experience. Introjects often lose their independent quality and become merged with one's sense of self, only to return later to their previous distance from the experienced self.

Imaginal dialogues may be spoken aloud (as in children's private or "egocentric" speech or in adults' solitude), written, or simply thought. When imaginal dialogues occur in speech, as is often the case with young children, one will observe the behaviors common to private speech: averted gaze, failure to make eye contact with any person present, distance maintained from the other, reduced loudness of speech (as contrasted to public speech) (Gallagher and Craig, 1978, 106). There is no protest from the child when a response is not forthcoming from a physically present other, since the speaker does not consider him or her to be the audience but rather the imaginal other to whom the speech was directed. There is often—though not always—manipulation of props (a doll, stone, finger) to represent the imaginal other. The imaginal dialogues of private speech—both speech used when alone and non-communicative speech when with others—can be differentiated from monologal private speech by the speakers implying an intended (imaginal) audience. Such an imagined audience can be indicated in a number of ways: by nonverbal actions or gestures (i.e., between two dolls), by change of voice or intonation, by direct reference to another, by specification of characters, or by utterance pairs which meet usual conversational constraints (i.e., question-answer, comment-acknowledgment pairs). If there is a sequence of utterances by a speaker, the conversational constraints of the first utterance are either met by the second utterance (double role dialogue),[1] or the second utterance presupposes that a response to the

---

[1] Example of double role dialogue: Here the child acts out first the role of the speaker and then the role of the listener-respondent. Rebecca (4;2) says the following as she plays on the floor with two boxes and wooden shapes of people and animals: (Child picks up a toy pig and has it bang on the box) "'Knock, Knock...' 'You're not coming in' [says the father doll]... 'All right I'll go back in my room...'" [says the pig] (Shields, 1979, 257). Example of single role dialogue: "(Child holding toy telephone to his ear) 'Hi.' (*pause*) 'No, I can't.' (*pause*) 'My mommy Holly.' (*pause*) 'Yes. Okay.' (*pause*) 'No.' (*pause*) 'Oh.' (*pause*)" (Gallagher and Craig, 1978, 108).

first has been imagined and not vocalized but has nevertheless served as a stimulus to the next spoken words (single role dialogue).

The choice of the term "imaginal dialogue" anticipates the point of view on the development of imaginal dialogues that will emerge in the course of this book. In using the word "imaginal" ("imaginal other," "imaginal dialogue") we follow Henry Corbin's (1972) distinction between the "imaginary" and the "imaginal." Corbin rejects the word "imaginary" when referring to these phenomena because in modern non-premeditated usage the "imaginary" is contrasted with the "real." "Imaginary" is equated with the unreal, the nonexistent. Our high valuation of the sensible world, the material and the concrete (what we take to be "real"), shines a pejorative light on the "imaginary." By using the term "imaginal," Corbin hopes to undercut the real-unreal distinction, and to propose instead that the imaginal not be assessed in terms of a narrowed conception of "reality," but a broader one which gives credence to the reality of the imaginal.

The word "dialogue" will be used here in two senses. First, it will be used to describe the literal process of exchange between two or more parties, whether it be verbal, gestural, or some combination thereof. Second, it will be used in Martin Buber's more limited sense as the goal of relatedness. For Buber not all verbal exchanges between two parties are dialogues; indeed true dialogue need not be verbal at all. According to Buber in true dialogue the integrity and autonomy of both self and other are preserved; one neither identifies with nor incorporates the other. Each can address and be addressed.

One finds imaginal dialogues across the life-span and in different life contexts: in children's play, in their conversation with their dolls and imaginary playmates, in adults' dreams and waking dreams and fantasy, in prayer, in authors' relations to their characters, in dialogues in private speech and thought, in literature and drama. Yet for the most part in psychology, these instances are treated separately. Here we will steal over the fences that have traditionally segregated private speech, play, imaginary companions, dreams, fantasy, prayer, the writing of novels and plays, the reading of literature, the viewing of drama...and thought itself. We do so not to pretend that there are no differences amidst these terrains, but rather to allow a different organization and differentiation of these experiences to challenge the theoretical explanations proposed for each singly. For, as we shall

INTRODUCTION 5

see, when each is treated singly, some curious theorizing emerges that for the most part sees imaginal dialogues as either disappearing or radically changing with age.

It is not enough for imaginal dialogues to suffuse the intimacy of our talk and thought. They need a conceptual space as well, where they can exist with integrity; a place in theory where their "development" is not reduced to a change from their presence in childhood to their absence in adulthood. They need a space in theory so we can ask, "Given their presence, their diversity, enduringness, and multiformity, what might their development entail?" Only when we have accepted their continued presence can we move closer both to describing the variations in their structures and to wondering at the multiplicity of their possible functions.

But to create this conceptual space we must first gradually free some area from the tangles of other claims. As we shall see some major developmental theorists would have us believe that, with age, imaginal dialogues should become transmuted almost entirely either to communication with "actual" others or to abstract thought. If we fully yield to these claims—focusing then on so called "real" dialogue or abstract thought—we lose the ground on which to argue for a different developmental course—one closer to the dramatic and imaginative thread that runs through them. There needs to be a space reserved in theory for imaginal activities; a space where they can be respected in their own right and not treated as merely ancillary or subordinate to other activities.

Any discussion of psychological function seems bound to operate within certain limitations. The researcher's vision of the world, of the course and endpoints of human development, determines the range of possible functions allotted to a phenomenon. Another researcher can dispute these proposed functions only by introducing new visions which are intended either to supplant or supplement the former. The difficulty of ascertaining the function of any single example of human speech or thought without a thorough knowledge of both the speaker and the context further complicates the effort to judge among proposed theories of function. And yet we cannot lay aside the question of function in despair if we wish to argue that human speech, action, and thought are not merely effects of previous causes. If we are to move beyond simply listing or describing what is, to penetrate the question of why it is so, then we are bound to the question of function. So we shall assume that imaginal dialogues are a means or a medium which serves certain ends.

When one speaks of the developmental course of a phenomenon, the question of function is always implicitly guiding the discussion. For instance if we view the function of imaginal dialogues as communication with literal others, then we will most likely construe such dialogues as "egocentric" speech, and hence as failed attempts at communication destined to be replaced by socially communicative speech as egocentricity diminishes. If, however, we assume the function of such imaginal dialogues in private speech to be self-communication, then we shall see these dialogues developing into internal speech, gradually changing form as the demands of self-communicative speech become differentiated from those of socially communicative speech.

One complication in examining imaginal dialogues and their development is that one has no grounds for assuming any single or unitary function that such dialogues might subserve. The possible functions are multiple, and the lines of development they suggest may not be convergent. Furthermore we will not have access to the simpler task often available in discussion of function—that of arguing against one proposed function while asserting another. The task we have set is more formidable: to work against the tendency to reduce imaginal dialogues to the set of functions proposed by the tradition of developmental psychology. While acknowledging much of the validity of the present claims in this area, we seek to reawaken another set of claims regarding function and thereby development. By looking at the implicit structures of the prevalent theories we shall gain a sense of the larger theoretical commitments which destine psychology's accounts of imaginal dialogues to be at best partial, at worst distorting.

For those clinicians who work with active imagination, play therapy, psychodrama, hypnosis, focusing, gestalt therapy, transactional analysis, the intensive journal method, psycho-imagination therapy, psychosynthesis, sandplay therapy, or guided imagery, this progression from theory to practice in this book may seem unduly slow, ready as you may be to embrace an interpretation of mind as dramatic. To quicken your patience, think of your colleagues who have seen your work as quackery, as encouraging split personality and hysterical dissociation, remember patients who were reluctant to converse aloud with figures from their dreams, fearful of "hearing voices." These popular therapeutic techniques do reflect the accessibility of imaginal dialogues for many people, but they lack an adequate grounding in developmental theory. Developmental theory, as we shall see, bears commitments which do not allow it to accept these (often hybridized) approaches. Although this text is rife with therapeutic implications—some consistent with one or another of the above mentioned approaches, some at odds[2]—it leaves the explicit consideration of psychotherapy to the end. Its major task is in clearing the ground for such work to become firmly rooted within a developmental psychology rather than remaining exiled.

As a reader you will be asked to ferret out the *dramatis personae* who inhabit your thoughts and actions—not only those of your childhood past, but those presently involved in conversation with you. Whatever your professional allegiance, I am purposely addressing the "developmental psychologist" within you first, and the "clinician" within you last. Too consistently psychology has given imagination over to the psychopathologists, fearful of the multiplicity of voices that do not simply appear in thought from time to time but that actually characterize thought.

Developmental psychology is not only practiced in departments of psychology, schools, and learning centers; it is practiced by each of us as we choose the forms of thought that we value most or least. Whether a developmentalist or not, we set about encouraging or rejecting certain kinds of speech and thought in ourselves and others, according to our theories (formal or informal) about their value. Whether or not we are students of developmental psychology, its theories have helped shape our developmental understandings as they have been practiced on us throughout our upbringing: by parents, schools, clinics, and by the culture at large.

---

[2] It is beyond the task of this volume to discriminate between the various therapeutic appraoches which acknowledge the multiplicity of the Self. Although some of their techniques appear similar, the underlying metapsychologies are often different, leading to conflicting views on the origin of imaginal others, their status in mind, and the therapeutic goal with respect to these figures. See Watkins' *Waking Dreams* (1974;1984, Chapters 3 and 4) for a critical differentiation of Jung's active imagination from various schools of guided imagery therapy.

If we are successful in our attempt to clear a conceptual space in psychology for imaginal dialogues (and perhaps through this example for other imaginal phenomena) and to underline a change in the direction of our talk about imaginal dialogues, then perhaps we will pause the next time we hear a child speaking with a doll, when we catch ourselves in dialogue with our critics, when we see someone praying. And in this pause, hopefully, will be a different sense of the possible futures of these moments.

PART I

Themes in Contemporary Psychological Approaches to the Functions and Development of Imaginal Dialogues

CHAPTER ONE

Imaginal Dialogues and Reason

Dictionaries remind us that reason, that "power of comprehending and inferring" associated with a "sane or sound mind," is "right thinking" (*Webster's*, 1960, 705), and some suggest that to think right is "to think logically" (*American Heritage Dictionary*, 1969, 1086). Nonetheless reason, or "right thinking," is not necessarily the kind of thought we each happily acquire over time, but a prescriptive and valuative notion of what thought should be like, ideally speaking. Developmental theorists are engaged as much as philosophers and poets in this prescriptive exercise. We have chosen three major developmental theorists—Piaget, Vygotsky, and Mead—to exemplify the effect of this prescribing exercise on theoretical notions concerning the development of imaginal dialogues. For in each case their observations and arguments about the functions and developmental course of imaginal dialogues, as different as they are, have been shaped by notions of reason, of what constitutes "right thinking." Other theorists could have been chosen. Our motive here, though, is not to comprehensively summarize theorists' propositions, but to explore how certain theoretical commitments have impacted our conceptions of imaginal dialogues.

That reason and imagination should be considered side by side is, of course, no novelty. Through the history of ideas they have struggled against each other, the winner fixing the light in which the other was seen. The particular question afoot, however, is how developmental theorists presently conceive of their relationship, and how this conception affects the discourse about imaginal dialogues.

Piaget

In Piaget's developmental psychology imagination and reason are most often seen as incompatible bedfellows, the latter pushing the former under the bed as ontogenesis proceeds. If imagination is seen as retained by reason it is taken only as subordinate to reason, not as intrinsic to it. This conception leaves imaginal dialogues in a vulnerable position—when present, destined to be superseded by, or transformed into, abstract thought; when absent, little cause for concern.

Piaget discusses imaginal dialogues in three contexts: in children's egocentric[3] speech, children's symbolic play, and adults' rehearsals of future conversations. Both egocentric speech and symbolic play are viewed pejoratively by Piaget for their failure in accommodation, or the child's adjustment to "reality."[4] Both are seen as symptomatic of the young child's profound egocentricity. Piaget approaches the imaginal dialogues of egocentric speech from the viewpoint of socialized speech, and those of symbolic play from the viewpoint of abstract thought.

One would expect Piaget to discuss imaginal dialogues in his volume, *The Language and Thought of the Child*. Here he differentiates all speech of the young child into two categories, egocentric speech and socialized speech:

> When a child first utters phrases belonging to the first group, he does not bother to know to whom he is speaking nor whether he is being listened to. He talks either for himself or for the pleasure of associating anyone who happens to be there with the activity of the moment. This talk is egocentric, partly because the child speaks only about himself, but chiefly because he does not attempt to place himself at the point of view of his hearer. (1955, 32)

---

[3] Piaget does not use the term "egocentric" in the colloquial sense of "self-centered," but in the cognitive sense of not differentiating one's own point of view from those of others, of not decentering.

[4] In Piaget's system, adaptation consists of a balancing between two processes: assimilation and accommodation. In assimilation the organism changes objects in its milieu in such a way that they can become incorporated into the structure of the organism. In accommodation, the organism adjusts itself to the demands of the object (Flavell, 1963). With respect to the child, a preponderance of assimilation over accommodation can be exemplified by play behavior, a preponderance of accommodation over assimilation by imitative behavior.

In drawing these distinctions, Piaget, as he later acknowledged (1962a), did not separate (a) speech incapable of rational reciprocity from (b) speech that is not intended for others. In his view the child always thinks he is talking to others and making himself understood.

So where would spoken imaginal dialogues fall in this division of child language? In his 1955 volume, Piaget offers only one example. A child addresses a tortoise and a salamander, as follows:

> "Now then, it's coming [a tortoise]. It's coming, it's coming, it's coming. Get out of the way, Da, it's coming, it's coming, it's coming... Come along, tortoise!"

> A little later, after having watched the aquarium, soliloquizing all the time: "Oh, isn't it [a salamander] surprised at the great big giant [a fish]!" he exclaims, "Salamander, you must eat up the fishes!" (39)

He uses this example to illustrate the child's primitive thinking, i.e., his attempt to command both animate and inanimate beings.

What are the positive functions allotted to the three kinds of egocentric speech Piaget addresses? Repetition or echolalia is seen as producing pleasure in talking in and of itself, without communicative intent. Monologues—in which the child talks to himself as though he were thinking out loud—are seen as marking the rhythm of, accelerating, supplementing, and sometimes supplanting actions. Finally, collective monologues "where an outsider is always associated with the action or thought of the moment, but is expected neither to attend nor to understand" are seen as creating the feeling that one is interesting to others (Piaget, 1955, 33). Piaget mentions in passing the way in which the child can "use words to bring about what the action of itself is powerless to do." An analysis of the role of egocentric speech in this "romancing and inventing," this "creating reality by words and magical language" (36-37) is not developed in this volume.

These few positive remarks, however, pale by contrast with Piaget's steady derogation of egocentric speech. The very name given to speech that does not have communicative impact on actual others—egocentric speech—is of course our first hint of what is to come. Piaget stresses how such speech reveals that "the child is constantly the victim of a confusion between his own point of view and that of other people" (1955, 39). The monologue is described as a "primitive and infantile function of language," of which "we shall naturally see the gradual disappearance...as we pass from early childhood to the adult stage" (40). When Piaget treats collective monologues, he compares them to the thinking aloud present in hysterical subjects. He sees the child's talking as failed communication—as "socially ineffectual"—because the child does not succeed in making his audience listen and because he is not really addressing himself to that audience. He is not speaking to anyone in particular. And though "he talks almost incessantly to his neighbors," the child "rarely places himself at their point of view" (60).

For Piaget this inadequate speech is reflective of the child's unsocialized thought. He parallels thought's change from egocentricity to "communicated intelligence" with speech's change from egocentricity to communicability. This comparison brings us to the one example Piaget gives of an imaginal dialogue in adulthood. Piaget mentions how an adult, when pursuing thought in an inquiry, imagines himself speaking with his "collaborators or opponents, actual or eventual, at any rate members of his own profession to whom sooner or later he will announce the result of his labours" (1955, 59). Piaget does not see this imaginal dialogue as a later development of the dialogues of egocentric speech, but contrasts the adult, who even in thinking is socialized, with the young child, who even in speaking is not; the adult, who even while alone thinks socially, with the child under seven who, even in the society of others, speaks egocentrically (60).

This theme of the inadequacy of the child's thought and its implicit impact on a consideration of imaginal dialogues can be further developed through an examination of Piaget's discussion of symbolic play in *Play, Dreams, and Imitation* (1962b). In this volume Piaget records many examples of imaginal dialogues in the context of symbolic play. As in his treatment of egocentric speech, he does attribute positive functions to these dialogues—once again, in an overall atmosphere of negative evaluation. He proposes that the child introduces an audience because she takes pleasure in imagining becoming the object of the other's attention. He further suggests that the child at times chooses to converse with an imaginary other rather than a real other because the imaginary other provides no resistance to the child's intentions or needs; there is no real other to accommodate to. Intentions and wishes are fulfilled with this release from the demands of accommodation. For Piaget such liberation is synonymous with pleasure. The dialogues are seen as part of the child's overriding desire to be the center of attention and to have reality conform to individual wishes. Traumatic interactions are also played out in these dialogues, with the implicit purpose of controlling or surpassing the particular life experience being represented. It is striking that although Piaget's chief claim for symbolic play is its role in cognition, the functions he ascribes are affective in nature and are presented without clear cognitive corollaries.

Piaget, while granting these positive functions to what we have called imaginal dialogues, has one eye on his conception of the intellectually developed adult as he scrutinizes the actions and speech of the young child. Symbolic play and its imaginal dialogues are considered a form of thinking, but an inadequate one where the "sole aim" is believed to be "satisfaction of the ego, i.e., individual truth as opposed to collective and impersonal truth" (Piaget, 1962b, 167). Piaget (1962a, 4) directly compares the child's thinking which is involved in the genesis of games to the "nondirected and autistic thought" Bleuler spoke of with regard to schizophrenia. This kind of thought, according to Piaget, wanes as the child becomes the socialized adult who is able to think abstractly—except in states of psychopathology. Imagining is seen as a "transitional moment in the development of the child's full cognitive capacities" (Casey, 1976b, 13). While the image is seen by Piaget as persisting in adulthood, its role in relation to conceptual thought changes radically: the image becomes merely a "symbol of the operational schema, and no longer as an integral part of it" (Piaget, 1962b, 244).

From Piaget's perspective the imaginal dialogues of egocentric speech develop into adequate communication with actual others. When imaginal dialogues are still present in adult speech, the adults who engage in them are described by Piaget as "certain men and women of a puerile disposition (certain hysterical subjects, if hysteria be described as the survival of infantile characteristics)" (1955, 40).

Vygotsky

Unlike Piaget, who sees egocentric speech as developing into communicative speech, Vygotsky sees it as developing from social speech. It is a stage in the development of inner speech, that is, in the inner verbalization of thought. For Vygotsky (1962, 43), thought and language arise independently, and only around age two do the curves of their development intersect with speech beginning to serve intellect and thoughts beginning to be spoken. Egocentric speech is seen by Vygotsky as "speech on its way inward." For Vygotsky (as for Mead) private speech is thus not an extension of the child's egocentrism, as it is for Piaget. Indeed, for Vygotsky the beginning of communication with oneself already presumed communicative ability and intent with others. He focuses on how the child begins to use speech to guide his own actions, to communicate with himself. Vygotsky comes to view such speech as not only accompanying activity, but as aiding in the direction, planning, and execution of action, and as serving mental orientation.

Although his is a more positive construal of private speech than Piaget's, Vygotsky also regards private speech as reflecting the young child's inabilities, i.e., to differentiate self-guiding speech from social speech, to differentiate self as auditor from other as auditor. As Kohlberg, Yaeger, and Hjertholm (1968, 969) point out, Piaget's and Vygotsky's viewpoints, while different, inevitably lead to a construal of private speech as "uneconomical and inefficient," having neither the economy of speech intended for self-guidance during performance of an action, nor the communicative value of speech intended for a differentiated other.

Vygotsky's interest is not in how thought preserves the dialogues of social discourse as a form with which to think, but rather how the form of speech used in communication to the other undergoes radical changes in structure as the function shifts to self-communication. He states: "While in external speech thought is embodied in words, in inner speech words die as they bring forth thought," "omitting the subject of a sentence and all words connecting with it," "leaving an elliptical, highly predicative syntax" (Vygotsky, 1962, 149, 139).

Vygotsky describes not only the decrease in quantity of egocentric speech with age (that Piaget also notes for different reasons), but a gradual change in its structure, such that by age seven egocentric speech looks radically different from social speech. According to Vygotsky, as egocentric speech is internalized, its structure shifts from dialogue to monologue. This is because the demands of self-communicative speech differ from those of both egocentric and social speech.

The one exception Vygotsky gives when inner speech approximates social speech in form is when inner speech prepares one for external speech, as when thinking over a lecture to be given. Vygotsky argues that predication is the natural form of inner speech because we "know what we are thinking about—i.e., we always know the subject and the situation" (1962, 145). Whereas in some social speech partners may be so intimate with each other's thoughts that predication alone is necessary for communication, Vygotsky claims that this is always so in inner speech. It is always so because in thought, for Vygotsky, speaker and auditor are always the same—namely, the self—and thus share the same knowledge of referents.

> In inner speech, the "mutual" perception is always there, in absolute form; therefore a practically wordless "communication" of even the most complicated thoughts is the rule. (145)

Thus for Vygotsky inner speech is necessarily monologal, and he claims that "psychological investigation leaves no doubt that monologue is indeed the higher, more complicated form, and of later historical development" than dialogue (1962, 144). The imaginal dialogues in children's private speech are seen as disappearing as speech becomes internalized and the more advanced monologal form is mastered. For Vygotsky,

> Dialogue implies immediate unpremeditated utterance. It consists of replies, repartees; it is a chain of reactions. Monologue, by comparison, is a complex formation; the linguistic elaboration can be attended to leisurely and consciously. (144)

Vygotsky compares the monologues of thought to the dialogues of social speech. He fails to compare the former monologues of thought to the dialogues of thought, an issue we shall explore in Chapter Four.

There appear to be three primary influences leading Vygotsky to hold monologic inner speech at the apex of verbal thought: the functions he ascribed to both egocentric speech and verbal thought; his implicit conception of the self as unitary; and his consequent lack of focus on the presence of imaginal others in thought. These topics will be taken up in Part II. For now, let us rest with seeing that the valued form of verbal thought, the monologue, which is elliptical and highly predicative, leads to an implicit view of imaginal dialogues in thought as inefficient and inferior.

Mead

For Mead, monologal thought does not hold a position developmentally superior to dialogal thought, as it does for Vygotsky. Nor does Mead, like Piaget, place imagination in opposition to reason. The imaginal dialogues present in children's play and speech are internalized without threat to reason. Indeed, from Mead's point of view, they are constitutive of reason, as thought for Mead is essentially dialogical.

While Piaget tends to see play and its imaginal dialogues as reflective of the autism of childhood, Mead sees such dialogues in play as reflective of the essentially social character of all psychical processes, those of children included. Thus, although Mead and Piaget would probably agree on some of the functions of such dialogues, Mead's commitment to the social nature of the self from infancy does not lead him to propose the disappearance of imaginal dialogues. These dialogues, rather than being construed as evidence of the child's inability to communicate with actual others or to deal with the demands of a social reality were for Mead—as they are for Vygotsky—evidence of exactly the opposite: the internalization of the social nature of reality.

Mead sees the child's early dialogues in play as gradually becoming the inner conversations of thinking. The dialogue as a form is central to Mead's thought, as he believed that it is through the reflexivity of the dialogue that the self arises. For Mead, all speech and thought are implicitly dialogical. The dialogue form establishes for the child the meaning of the self and her actions. Awareness of the self, according to Mead, arises through adopting the perspective of others toward oneself. This is achieved first through describing one's activities to another, or as though to another, and thereby evoking the response of the other to oneself. At first the self is the reflection of others' attitudes toward it. Thus, where Piaget's example of a child describing what she sees to her doll is taken by him to be expressive of the child's pleasure in being a focus of attention, for Mead this perpetual describing—which can strain the patience of those around children ("Now I'm putting on my hat. See me putting it on!")—marks the beginning of the child's transition to the role of the other, from which indeed one sees and becomes aware of oneself and others. As the child begins to take on all the roles of others toward oneself—policeman, parent, sibling, etc.—the child's own self is created. Indeed, for Mead, the self is an organization of perspectives. "When playing at being someone else, the self comes to realize its own nature at the same time it realizes the nature of the person whose role is being played" (Pfuetze, 1973, 83).

From this perspective, Mead argues that the importance of the novel and the newspaper is that they create the self by allowing the reader to adopt other perspectives. When one reads an "admirable novel…he feels in some sense enriched… His life has had content added to it. He has been given a new point of view, a new approach, a new way of looking at things; and the novelty involved in it leads to a richer experience…" (Mead, 1936, 410).

While Vygotsky argues that social speech and speech to oneself are essentially different in structure due to their divergence in function, Mead stresses the similarity between thinking and talking to somebody else. Thinking for Mead involves the ability to both assume one's own perspective, and to take the attitude of the group on it, being able to shift between these with ease.

> There is a field, a sort of inner forum, in which we are the only spectators and the only actors. In that field each one of us confers with himself. We carry on something of a drama. If a person retires to a secluded spot and sits down to think, he talks to himself. He asks and answers questions. He develops his ideas and arranges and organizes those ideas as he might in a conversation with somebody else. He may prefer talking to himself to talking to somebody else. (Mead, 1936, 401)

While Mead understands the dialogal form as persisting in thought once it is developed, he proposes that the nature of the interlocutor changes.

> Thus the child can think about his conduct as good or bad only as he reacts to his own acts in the remembered words of his parents. Until this process has been developed into the abstract process of thought, self-consciousness remains dramatic, and the self which is a fusion of

the remembered actor and this accompanying chorus is somewhat loosely organized and very clearly social. Later the inner stage changes into the forum and workshop of thought. *The features and intonations of the dramatic personae fade out* and the emphasis falls upon the meaning of the inner speech, the imagery becomes merely the barely necessary cues. But the mechanism remains social, and at any moment the process may become personal. (Mead, 1978, 180)

Whereas in childhood thought one speaks to specific others, in adulthood, Mead maintains, one usually converses in thought with a "generalized other." For Mead (1924-25) this transition from specific to generalized other, while never complete, is part of development "to the levels of abstract thinking and that impersonality, that so-called objectivity that we cherish" (272). The generalized other arises from the multiplicity of roles one has assumed in the past and appears to be a homogenization of these. It represents the attitude of the whole community, posing the hypothetical viewpoint of a "greater objectivity" against the "personal wants and attitudes" of the individual. Thus the function of this generalized other is the universalizing of thought (Mead, 1924-25, 90).

Finally, for Mead the transition from the multiple roles the child takes on in play to the unitary presence of the generalized other in adulthood reflects a more stable and mature development of self and, most importantly, is also seen as a development in thought. Although Mead does not characterize the dialogical form itself as at odds with "right thinking," his notion of good thought does lead him to propose a change in the nature and number of interlocutors in imaginal dialogues. The child's pantheon of particular presences who grace her play and fantasy, who join her in conversation, are seemingly reduced to one. The many names and faces, the particular intonations and voices merge, leaving a single voice, a homogenized unity.

CHAPTER TWO

Reality and the Imagination

In psychological theories imaginal phenomena—their origin, nature and functions—are most often approached through the measure of the "real." Imagination is seen variously as a rather dangerous and tricky opponent of the real, as little more than a mimic of the real, or as a help-mate to the real—always ready to rehearse for or react to moments of the real. In all three of these relations the real is understood as that which exists factually, actually, objectively (Morris, 1969, 1085-1086). It is the objectively verifiable reality of science that is given priority—i.e., that which yields to its methods. Perception, veridical memory, logical reasoning—acts which are defined as yielding "the real"—are set in opposition to imagining. Imaginal others and scenes are contrasted to "real" others and the material world, to that which is susceptible to the checks of consensual observation. As we shall see, these actual or "real" others are given clear ontological priority, with imaginal others usually derivative from and subordinate to them—suffused as they are with the untrustworthy stuff of "subjectivity."

In this chapter we will explore the three aforementioned relations between the real and the imaginary and their impact on conceptions about imaginal dialogues: the opposition of the imaginary and the real; the dependent, almost mimicking, relation of the imaginary to the real; and the imaginary as instrumental to one's relation to the real. To exemplify the first of these relations, we will explore psychoanalytic and Piagetian theories. To exemplify the latter relations, we will pursue Mead's social theory, as well as psycholinguistic and Russian psychological approaches.

The Opposition of the Real and the Imaginary

> ...a happy person never phantasies, only an unsatisfied one. The motive forces of phantasies are unsatisfied wishes, and every single phantasy is the fulfillment of a wish, a correction of unsatisfying reality. —Freud, 1907/1959, 146

> What is usually called fantasy disregards one or more aspects of reality, replacing them by arbitrary presuppositions; it is autistic. The greater the number of presuppositions and connections which do not correspond to reality, the more autistic the train of thought. —Bleuler, 1912/1951, 416-411

In many psychological theories the imaginary is placed in opposition to the real, as imagination is contrasted with perception. The real in such theories is decidedly more valued. Indeed, the imaginal acquires value only as it approaches a replication of the real. The products of imagination are most often seen as deformations or distortions of the real—distortions conceived in the service of wish, and created through such sleights of mind as condensation, substitution, and negation. The psychoanalytic and Piagetian psychologies both construe imaginal dialogues as forms of wish-fulfillment which are compensatory to the harshness of "reality."

Psychoanalytic Approaches

Just what is this real, this harsh reality that draws from us such intensity of wish that all manner of imaginal scenes and worlds are fashioned? Freud's answer is simply, but unequivocally, the external world:

> ...we are...confronted with the task of investigating the development of the relation of neurotics and of mankind in general to reality, and in this way of bringing the psychological significance of the real external world into the structure of our theories. (Freud, 1911/1957, 218)

For Freud the real is that "realm of obdurate fact as ruled implacably and without exception by the laws of natural science" (see Casey, 1971-1972, 663). In his theory reality has a harsh and hostile cast to it. The individual confronts it, but remains estranged from it (Casey,

1971-1972, 664). Indeed, the individual must confront reality from a defensive posture, viewing it as a source of deprivation and frustration. Out of this defense against reality arises the imaginal. In psychoanalytic theory, it is this tense opposition between the imaginal and the real that forms the very basis for discussion of both the functions and the developmental course of imaginal dialogues.

Of course, we must first account for the presence of imaginal others. These imaginal others have been discussed in the psychoanalytic literature as object representations, introjects, incorporated others, primary process presences, internalized others. In one carefully elaborated system, Schafer (1968) employs the term "primary process presences" to identify the broadly inclusive category of which "introjects" forms a subset. He proposes that these presences can be differentiated on the basis of how the subject experiences them spatially—as internal (introjects), external, or of indeterminate locality. Imaginal others or primary process presences are treated in psychoanalysis' technical discussions of hallucinations, children's play, imaginary companions, dreams and daydreams, and the vicissitudes of object relations.

These imaginal others are seen as the products of internalization, the assimilation of intersubjective relations into intrasubjective ones. Freud's (1940/1964) original example of this process was his description of the development of the superego:

> A portion of the external world has, at least partially, been abandoned as an object and has instead, by identification, been taken into the ego and thus become an integral part of the internal world. This new psychical agency continues to carry on the functions which have hitherto been performed by the people...in the external world: it observes the ego, gives it orders, judges it and threatens it with punishments, exactly like the parents whose place it has taken.(205)

Thus, originally the imaginal other is seen to be fashioned after actual others, in order to facilitate interactions with the external world. As attention to internalization grew in subsequent theorists' work, the figure of the superego was joined by others, and the self-regulatory function of the imaginal other was expanded upon.

These internal objects are contrasted with external objects as follows: whereas we are "vulnerable to the independent activity of the external object—to its abandoning, rejecting, punishing, demanding, traumatizing influences, and to its stimulating and gratifying influences too"—with the internal object one can minimize one's vulnerability to and maximize one's control over it (Schafer, 1968, 235). Thus some of the functions of internalization and its resulting imaginal figures are seen as enabling one to defend against reality and to seek security in an internal world where one has more control. Let us look at how psychoanalysis envisions the functions of relating to imaginal others. After this we can summarize the developmental courses prescribed for imaginal dialogues within this theoretical system.

Through relating to an imaginal other one can compensate for the absence or inadequacy of an actual other. Psychoanalysis proposes that the first object representation occurs as a hallucination of the absent breast, and later of the mother herself. When the child is confronted with an experience of a hostile or neglectful mother, a good mother may be imagined to compensate for the harshness of reality. Indeed this internal good mother may actually come to be preferred as the child experiences more of a sense of control over her; she does not present the same distressing fluctuations of mood and action as the real mother. Through imaginal dialogues one can not only supplement a deficient or discontinuous reality but, by reliving past traumatic situations and anticipating future ones, one can gain a sense of mastery and control over what in reality makes one feel weak, impotent, and inadequate.

In an imaginal dialogue the child can also interact with the voice of an adult to guide the child's actions, thus gradually liberating herself from reliance on external censors and punishments. In such superego-type imaginal dialogues, the child is able to play out her fantasy of omnipotent aggression while also personifying the restraining influence of a budding conscience—thus protecting herself from "the terror of her own omnipotent success" (Isaacs, 1933, 229). Through introjection and identification the child shares in the strengths and qualities of the other, thereby redressing the lack of equality in most child-adult relations. Thus in imaginal dialogues the child often identifies with the parent or adult, projecting onto her imagined partner her own usual stance as a vulnerable, needy, and often naughty child. Through such dialogues one gains distance and liberation from those qualities of self that are experienced as less desirable, while sustaining vicarious satisfaction through one's interactions with those in play and dialogue (Isaacs, 1933). This dramatic form allows different points of view to be tempered as well as expressed.

Object relations theorists (e.g., Klein, Fairbairn, Guntrip) maintain that just as one preserves the good self by isolating the bad self into a projection, one preserves the good aspect of the other by splitting those qualities of the real other experienced as good and as bad into separate personae. At an early stage of object representations, these two varieties of experienced qualities are most often isolated into different fantasy figures. This allows the child to preserve the good object and maintain a sense of security. An interesting thing about imaginal dialogues in play or daydreams is that the troublesome or "bad" aspects are not ignored or repressed, but are actively interacted with in the form of a dialogue while care is taken to protect the presence of good in self and other. Through the projection, introjection, and identification exhibited in such dialogues, the child has the power to change his psychological experience despite his powerlessness to influence his actual interactions with others. For example when the bad mother or father appears in play, the child often radically shifts the balance of power by introducing the figure of a policeman or a superhero who puts to rest the threatening behaviors of the bad mother or father.

Similarly through displacement from one object to another, less dangerous one, the child can vent his emotions without fear of retribution from the actual other for whom such feelings are felt. Aggressive fantasies, for instance, rather than being addressed to the father—who is bigger and more powerful, and on whom the child depends for support, love and approval—may be addressed in the form of an angry speech to a pretend robber. For further safety from feelings of powerlessness and fears of punishment for the expression of anger, he may imagine himself as a judge or Superman.

Through these mechanisms, as exhibited in the imaginal dialogue, the child is able to involve himself in the problematic feelings and aspects of his experience— but with the possibility of feeling a wholly different relation to them. The imaginal dialogue allows for a field of interaction between aspects of experience while leaving their presentation and resolution relatively unconstrained by the vicissitudes of reality.

Such functions implicitly describe an inner psychic world designed at first by wish where what one wants can be made to occur, as though one were godlike within the bounds of this province. This inner world is pitted against an outer world which is often felt as inadequate, discontinuous, hostile, overbearing, accusatory and punishing. With such descriptions the developmental directions proposed for imaginal dialogues are not surprising. The plurality of directions is intentionally emphasized here as psychoanalysis in its history and its present diversity of metapsychologies is far from unified regarding the fate of primary process presences. Nonetheless, some trends are widely—though not universally—shared.

It is ironic that Freud, a pioneer in presenting the reality of the psychological, should assert so forcefully the priority of the external and the material. Even after his proposal of psychical reality to account for how the strength of a fantasy of seduction might equal that of the actual experience of seduction, he retreated to suggest that perhaps such an actual seduction, though not present in the lifetime of an individual, had occurred to an ancestor (see Casey, 1971-1972, 677).

> It seems to me quite possible that all the things that are told to us today in analysis as phantasy—the seduction of children, the inflaming of sexual excitement by observing parental intercourse, the threat of castration (or rather castration itself)—were once real occurrences in the primeval times of the human family, and that children in their phantasies are simply filling in the gaps in individual truth with prehistoric truth. (Freud, 1917/1963, 371)

Freud's dichotomy between internal psychical reality and external, material reality was replicated even within the domain of the psychical as he ferreted out those representations that consensually converged with other people's and those that departed. Namely, due to his partial adherence to a copy theory of perception, he postulated that internal representations are of two kinds: those which reproduce external reality and those which are "drive cathected," which represent the psychical reality of the dreamer (Schimek, 1975, 174). The representations in dreams and psychosis, the "primary process representations," and those which appear to duplicate the objects of external reality were thus differentiated. The primacy afforded reality is shared with secondary process representations. Thus, development of object representations is most often seen not just as increasing the degree of complexity of characterization (i.e., from polarized representation—all good, all bad, etc.—to multidimensional representations), but as an increasing degree of correspondence between object representations and individuals in the external world.

At "primitive" levels of self and object-representation, characters are polarized—all good and idealized, or all bad and persecutory. Meissner (1981) describes the early polarized figures as organized along either aggressive or narcissistic lines. The former yield "aggressive" and "victim" introjects which are either powerful and destructive or vulnerable and helpless, while the latter yield "superior" and "inferior" introjects which are either replete with a sense of specialness, grandiosity, and omnipotence or with inferiority and worthlessness. Presumably as development progresses, "the alternation and interlocking of introjection and projection produce composite introjects" (Meissner, 1981, 22). The resulting images of self and other are more differentiated, "richer, more varied, more consistent and more congruent with what objects are really like" (Krohn and Mayman, 1974, 448).

The change from polarized to multidimensional characters is presumably made possible by a change in the structure of defenses. Klein (1975b) characterizes this transition as the one between the paranoid position and the depressive position. For instance as one moves from the primitive mechanism of splitting to ambivalence, representations change from all-good or all-bad to ones which are both accepting and rejecting, loving and hating. So as one can tolerate more of reality, there is a shift from wish-laden to realistic representations.

Rather than trace the full history of these genetic ideas within the work of various psychoanalytic theorists, we will turn our attention instead to a single psychoanalytic work, Schafer's *Aspects of Internalization* (1968), which attempted to summarize and critique these treatments. While proposing certain new ways of approaching the subject, Schafer conserves in his theory the basic psychoanalytic arguments regarding imaginal others and our dialogues and interactions with them. Schafer proposes a developmental continuum from primary process presences to secondary process object representations primarily along an axis of degree of congruence between actual person and representation of that person, between the psychoanalytic real and the imaginal. Whereas primary process presences, due to the suspension of a self reflective representation (i.e., an awareness that one is thinking), are felt in the moment of daydream as presences, in secondary process representation there is no longer the imaginal presence but merely the thought of another. Primary process presences are described as object representations which are "inaccurate, unstable and timeless due to the influence of unconscious motives and ideation," whereas secondary process object representations are "characterized by relative accuracy, stability, and a preserved temporal and spatial (external) index, and reflective processing" (126-127). "A reasonably faithful rendering of the object's pertinent essentials" (126), its essentials in reality, is contrasted with a distorted rendering, biased by wish and by unmitigated subjectivity. Thus development coincides with the imaginal's more accurate mirroring of reality and with a depersonification of presences.

On this last point Schafer is quite strict:

> Too often, introjects are written about (and discussed in the clinic) as if they are actual persons carrying on lives of their own, with energies of their own, and with independent intentions directed toward the subject. This is how patients often experience them and describe them, but is it good metapsychology? [...The introject's] seemingly independent ability to influence the subject is its outstanding experiential quality. (Schafer, 1968, 83)

Thus Schafer concedes that a language designed to reflect our phenomenological experience of these presences would speak of them as having thoughts, feelings, motives, and agency. Such a language, descriptive of experience, is not Schafer's concern. His is a language of efficient causal explanation. Given psychoanalytic theory, all thoughts, feelings and motives of an imaginal figure are referred back to the motives of the subject. They are "representations of the subject's wishes and conflicts" (Schafer, 1968, 138-139). Thus from Schafer's point of view, the primary process presence, even the "pejoratively colored persecuting introject is always doing what the subject tells it to do; its independent activity is only apparent" (139). For Schafer and other clinical theorists, development has to do with making experience conform to explanatory notions. Imaginal presences should in the end be experienced and "treated merely as the thoughts, ideas or information" (138) which theory says they are.

For Schafer the developmental question is "How does the introject lose its influence?... Put most broadly, the question is not, How is the irrational possible? but, How is the rational possible?" (136). With these considerations we reach a nexus in our discussions of reason and the imaginal, and reality and the imaginal. The irrational here is imaginal reality which diverges from external reality and the rational.

Schafer notes that "introjects" often recur without change. But rather than dealing positively with this stability of occurrence, Schafer understands it as the result of "strong, infantile, id-ego fixations...being represented by these dramatic personae" (139). From this point of view,

> ...introjects may be said to be instruments of the forces that oppose change; they must be assigned a mainly conservative role in the development of object relations...
>
> The specifically conservative or fixation aspect of the introject or any other presence is seen in its representing primitive or infantile basic assumptions and wishes concerning the relation of the subject to objects. (Schafer, 1968, 131-132)

Thus people who are predisposed to create introjects and other presences and to experience them repetitively are seen by Schafer as "dominated by infantile fixations," with "unremitting pressure of infantile wishes" and a "predilection for magical control over objects," all of which result in a "turning away from external object relations to fantasy" (132).

Schafer does not take up the issue of primary process presences that have no definite external referents—for example monsters, witches, and space people. Clinicians, beginning with Melanie Klein, have often seen the attaching of a worldly referent onto such figures as an indication of development. Thus Klein as a play therapist might, through interpretation, hope to have the child begin to treat the witch as mother, or the hungry naughty little pig as the child herself; again a redirection of the imaginal to the real.[5] Apropos our earlier discussion of the rational, Ekstein, a child analyst, attempts to befriend the patient's monster, talking directly to the "introject" in the session. His developmental goal is to introduce the monster to reason and

---

[5] In this regard see also Rambert (1949).

reflection via a relationship with the therapist. He wants the monster "to become someone with whom the patient and the therapist can negotiate," who can explain and create rationales for the patient: "the monster is changed in that he becomes more rational and subject to secondary process reasoning" (Ekstein, 1965b, 194).

As play is in psychoanalysis, imaginal dialogues are seen as a form of thinking which eventually changes into "secondary process reality-oriented thinking" (Ekstein, 1965a, 441). What results from this depersonification of thought is expressed variously by theorists. Some (such as Fairbairn) speak of an integration of imaginal egos, thus reducing their number and extending the bounds of the ego in this assimilatory project, while others, such as Kernberg, speak of how the imaginal others are integrated into the tripartite structure of id, ego, and superego. For Ekstein and others of the psychoanalytic persuasion, it is to be hoped that where "introjects ruled, capacity for object relations should be developed" (Ekstein, 1965b, 196-197).

One is reminded of the psychoanalytic literature on imaginary companions suggesting that the child who is in commerce with such companions is morbidly turning away from "real" others. Harriman (1937), for instance, wrote that imaginary companions result from a "temporary dichotomy" in one's personality and that "real playmates cause these fantasies to disappear" (368).

From the psychoanalytic point of view it would seem that were reality more adequate, imagination might cease to dream. But given the vicissitudes of reality, the very contrast and opposition between the imaginal and the real allows the ego a realm of rest from the world. In theories of play and daydreams this realm—when not taken to an extreme—is credited with making it more possible for one to "control his real behavior, and to accept the limitations of the real world"—to adapt. Dramatic representation "furthers the development...of the sense of reality. It helps to...enhance the child's readiness to understand the objective physical world for its own sake" (Isaacs, 1945, 210). Despite the fact that internalization is a necessary process both for the existence of an internal world and for interaction with the external world, psychoanalytic discussion of it is couched largely in terms of pathology. From the psychoanalytic perspective, the characters which result from internalization are representative of various infantile conflicts, corresponding to different stages of development and their characteristic defenses. Their origin is located in primitive, oral, sadistic, instinctual drives (Greens, 1954). The resulting introjects are seen in terms of narcissism and aggression. The young child is described as passing from a paranoid position to a depressive one. What a choice!

In adulthood, the characters (or representations) are often inferred from reported interactions and the quality of the transference neurosis. These inferred representations of self and other are rarely invited by traditional therapies to be experienced as felt presences. When they are so experienced spontaneously, they are seen as rivaling object relations or signaling a return to more primitive, infantile preoccupations.

We find the emphasis on adaptation to external reality central to Piaget's treatment of imaginal dialogues as well. Piaget's theoretical system rests on his notion of adaptation as an equilibrium between accommodation and assimilation. The imaginal dialogues in symbolic play reflect the child's unbalanced assimilation of reality to his own ego. Such imaginal experience does not reflect reality but distorts it. For Piaget (1971) the essential property of play is its "deformation and subordination of reality to the desires of the self" (339). Therefore for Piaget, development coincides with a change from such wish-fulfilling distortions of reality to play that becomes more and more adequately adapted to reality (as in the construction of games).

With regard to the ludic symbol, "progress in socialization," for Piaget (1962b), "instead of leading to an increase in symbolism, transforms play more or less rapidly into objective imitation of reality" (139). As egocentric assimilation becomes de-centered, "play becomes as much an expression of reality as an affective modification of it" (285). When games replace early symbolic play Piaget argues that their function is not to transport the child elsewhere, but to reproduce or continue the real world. The rise of games with rules is coincident with a decline in symbolism, the former being "progressively less distorting and more nearly related to adapted work" (140).

This direction is taken with respect not only to symbolic play but to imagination in general. Piaget places imagination under the rubric of "undirected" thought, in contrast to "directed or intelligent thought." This presumably undirected form of thought is not adapted to reality, says Piaget (1955), and creates for itself "a dream world of imagination; it tends not to establish truths, but so to satisfy desires, and it remains strictly individual and incommunicable" (63). For Piaget (1955) imagination's laws are not the laws of experience and logic but those of "symbolism and of immediate satisfaction" (63). Once again inadequate thought and unreality (or imaginal thought and the realm it gives birth to) are paired as an inferior syzygy, compared to "reason" and "reality."

Imagination as Derivative of and Help-mate to the Real

As we have seen, at certain moments theories emphasize the imaginal's distortion of the real. If any development is deemed possible, an increasing realism within the imaginal is advocated. At other times, the same theories (and others) stress the imaginal as an internalization of social reality. At first, internal representations of others may appear piecemeal and subject to distortion and inaccuracy. Gradually, however, the imaginal dimension of thought provides an internal stage on which past or future "real" events—events of the external world—may be replayed or rehearsed in service of one's adaptation to reality.

For Mead imaginal dialogues, like thinking itself, result from an internalization of a social reality. The imaginal is derived from the real and remains in the service of the real, for the purpose of adjustment to the real. Like Piaget's example of an adult preparing his ideas in thought before an imaginary audience of colleagues or critics, Mead too sees inner conversations as a means of testing and rehearsing alternative solutions before one acts in reality. For Mead the imaginal dialogue is never just a mental process which exists wholly apart from action in the social world.

> He takes different roles. He asks questions and meets them; presents arguments and refutes them. He does it himself, and it lies inside of the man himself. It has not yet become public. But it is a part of the act which does become public. We will say he is thinking out what he is going to say in an important situation, an argument he is going to present in court, a speech in the legislature. That process which goes on inside of him is only the beginning of the process which is finally carried on in an assembly. It is just a part of the whole thing, and the fact that he talks to himself rather than to the assembly is

simply an indication of the beginning of a process which is carried on outside. (Mead, 1936, 402)

Theologically minded colleagues and students of Mead's brought to his attention the similarities between his conceptions of the generalized other and conceptions of God. But Mead is adamant in his rejection of such a notion, adhering to social reality, the individual voices and one's generalization of these, as the only reality which the imaginal can reflect.

One of the richest compendia of imaginal dialogues in early childhood can be found in the psycholinguistic literature. For the most part psycholinguists have seen these dialogues as "imitations of communication" (Slama-Cazacu, 1976), through which the child gains practice for actual communication with real others. Slama-Cazacu, in her book *Dialogue in Children* (1976), describes these dialogues as "surrogates of communication, compensatory forms of dialogue" (35) which occur primarily when there is no real other for the child to interact with. Again the priority is the real other; the imaginal is only second best. Weir, in *Language in the Crib* (1962), sees imaginal dialogues as similar to doing grammatical exercises or instructing oneself in a foreign language. George Miller corroborates this view, proposing that "only the pleasure of increased competence could have served as a reward" for this "self imposed drill—a playful drill, admittedly—that must serve to bring what he already knows up to a level of complete automaticity" (quoted in Weir, 1962, 15). Gallagher and Craig (1978), in their research on structural characteristics of imaginal dialogues, end up seeing the function of such dialogues in private speech (what they call "monologic conversations") similarly to Weir, i.e., as "highly structured means by which the child explores semantic and conversational language categories" (116). Thus imaginal conversations are mere imitations of "real" conversations for the purpose of increasing one's competence in "real" dialogue.

Just as Vygotsky conceived of egocentric speech and its dialogues as instrumental in planning and executing actions in the external world, later Russian psychologists conceived of imagination as "the ability to form new representations on the basis of previous experience, which allows for the planning of future actions"; it is a "creative reflection of reality" (Repina, 1971, 255). In their treatment of the development of imagination, Russian psychologists give clear and consistent priority to external, social, material reality. Novel images are seen as restructurings of previous experiences. The "observed richness of imagination" and images which depart from a focus on realism are seen as signs of weakly developed critical thinking, of "an inability to differentiate the possible from the impossible," and of a lack of knowledge about "what and how things exist in reality" (Repina, 1971, 255-256, 260). On the one hand then, the child is seen as innately concerned with realism, rejecting elements in fantasy that do not correspond to material and social reality. But on the other hand, this realism is taught to the preschooler:

> The realism of a child's imagination requires an active upbringing. It is imperative that the child's imagination be developed in connection with enriching his experience by knowledge of reality, and that it not turn into an unfruitful fantasy that serves as an escape from reality. (Repine, 1971, 261)

Imagination is to remain linked to action in the material world. At the end of the preschool period, the child can imagine without acting, but this imagining is to function as a plan for action, i.e., to guide or regulate future actions in the material world.

Although Russian psychologists have criticized Western approaches to the imaginal as idealistic and bourgeois (Repina, 1971), and as lacking an appropriate emphasis on reality, this is hardly the case—even in the primary object of their critical attack, psychoanalysis.

Freud painstakingly plotted out ways in which the imaginal was derived from the real, tracing dreams back to day residue, representations to perceptions, and fantasized scenes to actual events (ancestral or otherwise). Side by side with psychoanalytic concern about the imaginal as a flight from reality, we also find acknowledgment of the ways in which the imaginal prepares one for reality. For Hartmann (1939) fantasy can be seen as a regressive detour on the way to adaptive action, in that it allows one to plan. Schafer (1968) describes many daydreams as representational in a "down-to-earth, realistic, fashion."

> [They] may faithfully represent adaptive means-ends relations: communication may use organized speech and conventional gestures; action may observe the modes and

> limits of space, time, and bodily organization; and so forth. These details of the daydream may be no different from those involved in realistic planning. They may represent what is conceivable according to the reality principle. (89)

Schafer also describes how experience with hostile introjects helps a person acquire "aggressive skills" which may have a "wide range of utility" (1968, 132). For Peller (1954) the imaginal dialogues of play, in addition to all their wish-fulfilling functions, also prepare the child for adult roles. And Erikson proposes that in play the child creates model situations in which he can begin to "master reality by experiment and planning" (1950, 195).

Thus in psychoanalytic theory imaginal dialogues, like daydreams in general, are placed along a continuum according to function. The proposed functions range from escaping reality and fulfilling wishes (images as distortions of the real), to replicating the real and helping one adapt to reality in a straightforward manner (images as approximations of the real). From this perspective the phantasies of art are merely "precious reflections of reality" (Freud, 1911, 224), their only value to return us to external reality (Casey, 1971-1972, 678-679). As Casey has aptly summarized Freud's theory:

> Either we confuse psychical reality with [external] reality, as in dreams and psychosis; or the two types of reality are essentially similar as in neurosis and art. In neither case is psychical reality allowed to constitute a truly autonomous realm...its constituents are derivative from and thus dependent upon the material realm: psychical reality is in the end more the shadow of external reality than its equal. (674)

CHAPTER THREE

Seeing Imaginal Dialogues as Primitive

In the previous chapters we discussed exemplars of a variety of psychological approaches to imaginal dialogues. Our presentation was organized to highlight the fact that those approaches tend to describe and evaluate imaginal dialogues in terms of certain ontological commitments (i.e., the real is the tangible, the publicly shared, the socially agreed upon, and the secular) and axiological commitments (i.e., logical-scientific reasoning and socialized communication are the apices of developmental progress). In the context of such commitments and presuppositions, imaginal dialogues are envisaged in children as either (a) an early and surpassable stage in the development of abstract thinking; (b) as an early and surpassable stage in the development of communicative speech or socially shared reference to reality; or (c) as an early and surpassable stage in the adequate conceptualization of other "real" people.

These assumptions yield a set of specific (yet often contradictory) developmental expectations for imaginal dialogues. Viewed as an early stage in the development of abstract thought, the imaginal dialogues of private speech are seen as being progressively internalized. In the process either their structure becomes monological rather than dialogical, or the interlocutor becomes a generalized other rather than a specific other. Viewed as an early stage in the development of communicative speech, the imaginal dialogues of private speech supposedly become increasingly elaborated according to the demands of a "real" listener, such that the presumed "egocentric" qualities fade, allowing such speech to be understood by a "real" other. Finally, when imaginal dialogues are viewed as an early stage in the development of adequate conceptions of "real" people, the imaginal others of such dialogues are presented to undergo a radical change of character, from superficial and one-sided to multidimensional; from fantastical creations to copies of people in the subject's ideal interactional world.

Given these predictions, the persistence of imaginal dialogues in adults is taken either to reflect immaturity and pathology or to subserve the function of rehearsal for future social interactions. These ways of regarding imaginal dialogues may easily incline educators who are influenced by psychological theories to inhibit the public manifestation of such dialogues in public—seeking to curtail or eliminate "primitive and immature" behavior patterns. This is the case in Polish nursery schools where children are forbidden to talk to imaginary companions or to themselves when they could be speaking with "actual" people (Slama-Cazacu, 1976). It is commonly hoped by professionals and lay people alike that children's imaginal others will be quickly replaced by "actual" peers. Imaginal dialogues, like daydreams, are thought to be asocial, a turning away from reality. As such, they are seen primarily as an escape from the demands of consensual validation of reality, which communication with "real" others ostensibly promotes. From these perspectives daydreams and imaginal dialogues are held to be expressive of the "autoeroticism, egoism, and passivity" of the subject, of "uncluttered and unhampered egocentricity" (Schafer, 1968, 87-88). The popularity of psychiatric literature on so-called "split personalities" has reinforced the assumed correlation between the experience of multiple voices in thought and severe pathology. All this has caused the studying of imaginal dialogues in adulthood to be dismissed, except as a means of examining primitive forms of cognition.

Although hallucinations will be discussed at greater length in Chapter Eleven, the reduction of all imaginal dialogues to the status of hallucinations and archaic states must be briefly mentioned here. Perhaps no work has so eloquently consigned imaginal dialogues to the realm of primitivity as Julian Jaynes' *The Origin of Consciousness in the Breakdown of the Bicameral Mind* (1976). This fascinating and compelling book compares the voices heard by the Iliadic heroes and Joan of Arc, to those of present day schizophrenics. It explores the similarities among the imaginal dialogues of religious and mythic experience, of poetic experience, and of psychopathology. The propensity to hear voices is explained by what Jaynes calls a bicameral structure of mind,[6] which was pervasive among the "primitives" of 3000 years ago and can be found in "primitive" states in the present (such as schizophrenia).

Jaynes argues that in the past men would speak to their "gods" whenever a novel decision had to be made. No sooner had they heard the voice of the god than they followed its advice or command through action. This was so, he maintains, until the second millennium B.C.E.— a time of war, natural catastrophe and mass migrations. Survival under these conditions required a shift away from bicameral consciousness. One now needed to be able to postpone or even bypass obedience to the god's voice in order to survive an immediate external threat, as the god's advice was often no longer suited to the rapidly changing circumstances. People had to develop a subjective sense of themselves which could be different from how they displayed themselves to an enemy. In other words they needed the ability to appear to others differently from how they thought and felt.

Essentially what I shall call "the dialogical structure of mind" is understood by Jaynes as being based in the physiological and biochemical properties of the brain. Presumably the left hemisphere produces the voice which is heard by the right hemisphere, as the message is transmitted over the anterior commissure. In times of stress there is a buildup in the blood of the breakdown products of adrenaline, which lowers the threshold for such occurrences of voice.

Jaynes maintains that in ancient times, owing to a lack of consciousness (as we know it), stress was felt each time a decision had to be made that could not be dealt with by force of habit. In modern

---

[6] It is not surprising that the more the study of the brain has advanced, the more the realm of hearing voices is subsumed under discussions of brain function, attempting to explain the imaginal in terms of organic substrata. An interesting precursor to Jaynes' theory of bicameral consciousness was Leuret's work. Leuret (1834) attempted to explain the physiological basis for psychotics' conversations with their hallucinated figures. He argued that each part of the patient's twofold nature—self and imaginal other—resided in one of the two hemispheres of the brain. Leuret abandoned his explanation when confronted with psychotics who conversed with several voices!

times a reversion to a bicameral mind is experienced by those unfortunate individuals who cannot excrete the adrenaline by-products of stress as quickly as the rest of us.

Jaynes (1976) treats the functions of these internal voices much like the other theorists we have discussed: as voices which initiate and guide behavior, as "authority figures created by the nervous system out of the patient's admonitory experience and his cultural expectations" (411). Narrowing the function of imaginal dialogues to the initiation and guidance of behavior restricts the kinds of voices and figures Jaynes can deal with (admonitory and authority figures) and the kinds of response made to them (obedience.) What were once experienced as gods, Jaynes argues, are now called hallucinations. They are no more than certain "organizations of the central nervous system" (74). Jaynes sees the schizophrenic as one "waiting on gods in a godless world" (432).

It may be that the dialogical structure of mind has some basis in anatomy and biochemistry. What is of particular interest here, however, is the developmental argument advanced by Jaynes; namely, that imaginal dialogues are early and surpassable stages of thought, except in cases of psychopathology.

Are schizophrenics prone to a biochemical problem that the rest of us have evolved out of, leaving them with the figments of gods, and us with the relative silence of monologal, abstract thinking? Or is Jaynes' theory an expression of our cultural *Zeitgeist* confining the figures of imagination to primitive times and states of pathology, reducing their origin to the physiological and the biochemical? Jaynes himself speaks eloquently about the progressive secularization of our culture that has culminated with the present stage of modern science.[7] However, instead of reading his own theory as part of this sociocultural movement toward the "scientific"—that is, toward the

---

[7] Those familiar with Jaynes' work will no doubt notice as this book progresses the similarity of sources and phenomenological observations, particularly *vis à vis* the problematic aspects of some hallucinations: the authoritarian structure of relation between self and imaginal other, the reflexive obedience to the voice, the absence of an observing, narrating self who can distance from the voice's commands. Though Jaynes agrees that not all hallucinations are problematic, those that do not fullfil the above- mentioned structure while posing a challenge to his theory as to the functions and causes of voices are not dealt with convincingly. Despite this, there is hardly better reading than Jaynes' volume for those on the path toward understanding the nature of theories dealing with imaginal dialogues.

secular and the physical—he assimilates the movement into his theory. There is a progressive secularization as the culture moves away from the bicameral mind.

Let us at least entertain the reverse notion: that with increasing secularization, cultural conventions and "scientific" theories (Jaynes' among them) arise which discourage and disparage the experience of imaginal dialogues. As the prevailing scientisms erode our previous understanding of these voices—as issuing from divine entities—they attempt either to eliminate the experience of voices altogether; to confine the experience to childhood, or else to relegate it to the realm of the pathological, that which the culture would like to discard.

In large measure the prevailing developmental approaches addressed here have gained credence because imaginal dialogues of a public kind do seem to disappear with age. For those developmental theorists who take changes in age as the best index of developmental advance, the apparent cessation of public self-talk would seem to indicate that such imaginal dialogues are "primitive phenomena" that are replaced or superseded either by purely monologal thought or by socially directed, socially adequate communication with real others. In sum, imaginal dialogues are taken to be transformed into (or replaced by) wordless thought or articulated and responsive interchange with "real" others.

That the ostensible decline in imaginal dialogues with age (in adolescence and adulthood) might be due to social factors—more specifically, social taboos—is rarely if ever considered by development theorists, especially those who are inclined to see earlier forms of action and interaction "replaced" by chronologically later ones. That there may be no real decline in imaginal dialogues, either historically across cultures or ontogenetically—that they may continue throughout history and throughout the life of an individual (even in "normal" and "superior" adults)—would undercut the "transformation" argument. But what if this were indeed the case ? What if imaginal dialogues continued to flourish side by side with abstract thought and socially directed communication?

Forms of Talk (1981), by the sociologist Erving Goffman, may serve to expose the conspiracy of scientific and conventional silence surrounding "self-talk." By describing precisely the occasions when one engages in self-talk and when one does not, Goffman challenges the developmental theories which see the appearance of such talk in adult life as pathognomic or as a sign of immaturity. He insists instead that these theories, while pretending to scientific impersonality, actually reflect and sustain social conventions.

When we are left alone, Goffman (1981) reminds us to admit, do we not

> have occasion to make passing comments aloud? We kibitz our own undertakings, rehearse or relive a run-in with someone, speak to ourselves judgmentally about our own doings (offering words of encouragement or blame in an editorial voice that seems to be that of an overseer more than ourselves), and verbally mark junctures in our physical doings. Speaking audibly, we address ourselves, constituting ourselves the sole intended recipient of our own remarks. Or, speaking in our own name, we address a remark to someone who isn't present to receive it. (79)

People implicitly agree either to attend to each other's speech or to pretend to attend. To speak aloud to an imagined other in the company of "real" others is a breach of this agreement, for in addition to displaying that our attention is elsewhere, it demands by the terms of this reciprocal arrangement and by the very nature of talk, that our inner concerns be attended to by people to whom we are not attending. We know that as long as we appear to be attending we may speak with whomever we prefer in the privacy of our thought. But let these private conversations become audible and eyes begin to turn our way with disdain as well as fearful curiosity.

Goffman adds weight to his "interactional approach" by looking at instances when self-talk is considered appropriate, even required, in social situations. He argues for the sophistication of such talk, for without written rules and without having been told which social contexts require or permit it, we have learned well when self-talk is called for. Do we not all recognize the following situations?

> 1. You are walking down the street and you trip. You are aware that others are watching you. Do they wonder if you are drunk, clumsy, or daydreaming? You re-establish your reputation by showing that you have noticed yourself tripping. You examine what might have caused it (implying that anyone walking this way would have tripped), and then you "utter a cry of wonderment, such as, *What in the world!*" (Goffman, 1981, 90).

2. You are giving a talk and your notes are disarranged. You begin self talk: *Oh, my, they were here just a minute ago... Now, why can't you find them... Just a minute... Be calm*—something to let the audience know that some part of you is "shocked by the hitch and in some way not responsible for it" (92).

3. In the absence of praise or criticism from another, you verbalize it yourself, aloud, as though it were coming from someone other than yourself: *Now, George, that was a very good job, man. Very good, indeed!*

4. When you are fearful that another may think you are malingering or fooling about, you begin to annotate your behavior: *I am picking up these things, taking them upstairs, then...*

5. You are free to sing to yourself in the shower; or

6. Talk to yourself aloud in the car when alone.

In short in the privacy of our studies, our bathrooms, and our cars, or on our walks in nature, do not our very utterances betray that although there is but one actor literally present, there are often at least two roles? Why, argues Goffman, if we are all aware of this fact, do our theories continue to attribute such behavior only to adults of "puerile disposition" or "hysterical" nature (Piaget, 1955, 40)—to egocentric people or social isolates? Goffman attributes the familiar developmental interpretation of self-talk to the societal taboo against such talk. If we could set aside this taboo, Goffman argues, we would find that the more illuminating approach to such discourse is not the ordinary developmental one but rather an interactional one. Why the taboo? To speak to an imaginal other or to oneself in the presence of actual others is a situational impropriety because it is experienced by those actual others as a threat to intersubjectivity. In other words "reality" is that which we share; it does not include private conversations between self and imaginal others. We need only think of Jimmy Stewart's difficulty being loyal to Harvey in the presence of others!

If children exhibit self-talk more regularly than adults, it is not simply because they fail to make crucial distinctions (such as between speech for oneself and speech for others), or because they are prone to autism and egocentricity. It is rather because they have learned their lessons from adults well. As Goffman (1981) explains,

> George Herbert Mead notwithstanding, the child does not merely learn to refer to itself through a name for itself that others had first chosen; it learns just as early to embed the statements and mannerisms of a zoo-full of beings in its own verbal behavior...
>
> [By using] a lisping sort of baby talk, the parent makes it apparent that it is the child that is being talked *for*, not to. In addition, there are sure to be play-beings easy to hand—dolls, teddy bears, and now toy robots—and these the parent will speak for, too. So even as the child learns to speak, it learns to speak for, learns to speak in the name of figures that will never be, or at least aren't yet, the self. (150-151)

We teach children to engage in such fanciful and self-dissociated discourse with their dolls, fire engines, toes and fingers. We reward these behaviors with our amusement and obvious enjoyment. Perhaps we enjoy vicariously a freedom of expression denied to adults by social convention.

These kinds of self-talk, far from being evidence of primitivity, can be seen as the achievement of rather sophisticated abilities. For Goffman, early self-talk anticipates the essentially "theatrical" nature of adult speech, where one takes on accents, adopts the intonations of others, imbeds quotations both in discourse and in writing, and where, as we have seen, one is privileged to speak for dogs, babies, and objects. As adults we can "refer to earlier selves," and "convey words that are not our own," using adages to corroborate our own words with an anonymous authority other than ourselves (Goffman, 1981, 150). For Goffman, unlike Vygotsky and Mead, the internalization of self-talk is not necessarily a developmental advance. It may be seen, rather, as a reflection of the child's growing awareness of societal taboos. Thus self-talk does not disappear entirely with the arrival of abstract thought or the demands of socially shared discourse, but only limits the occasions of its appearance as rules of interaction shift with age. It does not pass away, but confines itself to those contexts where it is not censured. Thus, Goffman proposes,

> Instead, then, of thinking of self-talk as something blurted out under pressure, it might better be thought of as a mode of response constantly readied for those circumstances in which it is excusable. (1981, 96)

We would argue that the taboo against imaginal dialogues in private speech results not only from people demanding our display of interpersonal attention, but from conventions regarding the nature of reality, rationality and the idea of development. These conventions have encouraged either a global dismissal of imaginal dialogues (especially adult ones), or their subsumption into other discussions (of private speech, play, development of abstract thought or social discourse).

Imaginal dialogues represent not only a breach of our agreement to pretend to be listening to actual others, but also frequently a breach with a secular view of reality which holds that one's conversations are not to be peopled by gods, angels, muses, gnomes or other strange characters. They also constitute a breach with a unitary concept of the self that relies on a stable identity and does not look closely at shifts of mood, tone, or attitude that might suggest a multiplicity of the self. When we are granted partners in thought, they have been secularized not only in function but in identity—the imaginal voices have been returned to known others or aspects of self.

We are reaching for a perspective from which the development of imaginal dialogues is no longer entangled with chronology and ontogenesis (Kaplan, 1959), where the structures of imaginal dialogues are understood with respect to their own functions rather than set against the goals of either abstract thought or actual social discourse, and where "development" is not equated with a transition from the presence of such dialogues to their absence. To propose other ways of conceiving of the development of imaginal dialogues, we must first free ourselves from our usual notions of reason, reality and development—for as we have seen, these notions have been fundamental in shaping theory and research around imaginal dialogues. To this end, let us proceed with Part II of our study.

PART II

A Critique of Contemporary Psychological Approaches to Imaginal Dialogues

CHAPTER FOUR

Imaginal Dialogues and Reason

Come...let us reason together. —Isaiah 1:18

[Thinking is] the dialogue of the soul with itself. —Plato

[Imagination is] reason in her most exalted mood. —Wordsworth

The *Greater Hippias*, purportedly by Plato, sets the stage for imaginal dialogues to be seen as fundamental to reason. It is about what happens when we come home to ourselves. When Hippias, a rather thickheaded man, goes home at night he remains by himself. This is not only because he lives alone, but because "he does not seek to keep himself company. He certainly does not lose consciousness; he is simply not in the habit of actualizing it" (Arendt, 1971, 188).

In contrast, when Socrates goes home, he is met by a voice: "a very obnoxious fellow who always cross-examines him" (Arendt, 1971, 188). Socrates describes this fellow as follows:

> He is a very close relative of mine and lives in the same house, and when I go home and he hears me give utterance to those opinions he asks me whether I am not ashamed of my audacity in talking about a beautiful way of life, when questioning makes it evident that I do not even know the meaning of the word "beauty"[...]
> And yet, he goes on, how can you know whose speech

is beautiful or the reverse—and the same applies to any action whatsoever—when you have no knowledge of beauty? And so long as you are what you are, don't you think that you might as well be dead? (Plato, 1961, 1559)

Socrates wants to come to some agreement with his relative, to become friends with this voice; after all, they must live under the same roof. Hippias avoids this voice by ceasing to think, by refusing to open a dialogue.

Here dialogue is synonymous with internal dialogue; in Plato's words, thought is that "voiceless colloquy of the soul with itself." When we come home to ourselves, we can either invite the inner voices or disregard them—although sometimes, of course, they come uninvited, taking us deeper into the perplexities and complexities of an issue. Despite our familiarity with these voices of thought, many of our theories derogate this imaginal multiplicity, pitting reason against imagination, separating reason from its roots in argument and discussion with another, such as in dialogue.

Before we return to our colleagues Piaget, Vygotsky, and Mead, let us pause for a few moments outside of this century and the contemporary discipline of psychology to look at the ways in which relations between imagination and reason have been conceived of in other times and places. From this distance we shall be able to see that neither the modern divorce of imagination from reason nor the subordination of imagination to reason are intrinsic and inescapable facts of development, impartially described.

In a recent study on imagination, the philosopher Edward Casey (1976b) observes that, throughout the history of philosophy, imagination has been cast by thinkers into three main roles: imagination as subordinate to other faculties, where images are only imitations of imitations (Plato); imagination as mediator between perception, sensation and intellect (Aristotle, Hobbes, Kant); and imagination as superordinate to all human faculties including reason itself (German Romantics). Each of these views, dissimilar as they are, reveal in common a failure to acknowledge what Casey (1976b) calls the "multiplicity of the mental," a multiplicity which would preclude any rigid hierarchical structure among faculties (19). Abandonment of the effort to form a hierarchy, in which one favored faculty reigns in one century, only to be deposed in the next, would result, Casey holds, in a conception of imagination as "nonderivative, as a phenomenon to be evaluated on its own terms" (19). When applied to imaginal dialogues, this conception would lead us to approach actual instances of imaginal dialogues with the expectation of finding a multiplicity of relations among imagining, remembering, feeling, knowing, and sensing. Were all instances of imagining to be forced because of a *prejuge du monde* into a single continuum of value, the multiplicity would be falsely narrowed and homogenized.

Such homogenization is indeed what we find in the writings of Piaget, where formal operations are undoubtedly given a privileged position in the totality of functions. Kaplan (1983b) wonders,

> Is it possible that what Dewey calls an "occupational psychosis" has led many "cognitive-developmental" psychologists to presuppose formal operations or intelligence as *the* telos of development, and to represent ontogenetic changes solely in terms of those actions-instrumentalities pertinent to logical thought? (66)

Piaget, in his concern with the development of communicative language and formal-operational thought, lets imaginal dialogues fall between the rigid fingers of his arguments and preoccupations. He uses what he calls "egocentric speech" as one kind of evidence to support his claims about the child's intellectual immaturity, or egocentricity. It was his intention to demonstrate a gradual development from the child's egocentric stance to the adult's ability to decenter. Therefore he characterizes the young child's imaginal dialogues negatively. They are taken principally as evidence of incapacity. The young child is described as being unable to fully differentiate self as speaker from the other as auditor; unable to take into account the listener's viewpoint; and unable to construct speech adequate to the goal of communicating. The child, in speaking, does not collaborate with an audience or evoke a dialogue from the other. Interestingly, when Piaget in *Play, Dreams, and Imitation* (1962b) turns his attention to play, bountiful examples of imaginal dialogues are given. This is in contrast to his single example in the earlier work on language and thought (1955).

If, as is apparent, Piaget from the outset observed and recorded numerous examples of imaginal dialogues, why did he not use these to extend his notions of the functions and forms of egocentric speech?

It would seem most plausible to assume that Piaget's interest in the development of the socially adapted individual led him to construe egocentric speech primarily as failed communicative language. Had Piaget looked at imaginal dialogues in his work on children's speech with a less monolithic focus, his insistence on the child's profound egocentricity would doubtless have been called into question. One can see what might have taken place if one considers Shields' (1919) study of nursery-school children. In her observations of the children's private speech during doll-play, she found many instances of dialogues in which the child alternated between two or more viewpoints. These conversational sequences were as long as actual dialogues. They shared the features of actual dialogues (address, turn-taking, speech-act cohesion), and actually carried more referential material than one would have expected, given the claim that the speech of the young child is highly elliptical and abbreviated in form (Shields, 1979, 259).[8]

The same kinds of imaginal dialogues in children's play that Piaget takes as evidence for the child's egocentrism can be seen—and were indeed seen by the Romantics—as the initial steps in freeing oneself from a self-centered world. In pretending to be another and in engaging in imaginal dialogue with imaginal others, the child, like a young Proteus, breaks free of the bonds of a narrowly construed identity. Piaget, of course, has elsewhere stressed the value of the child's ability to change perspectives, but he fails to do so when he reports on his daughter playing the part of mother toward her doll.

It seems that since imaginal dialogues could not be presented as unequivocal manifestations of children's egocentrism, Piaget ignored them in his discussion of children's speech. This being the case, one must question the relevance for imaginal dialogues of Piaget's (1955) predictions for the fate of egocentric speech:

> But as we pass from early childhood to the adult stage, we shall naturally see the gradual disappearance of the monologue, for it is a primitive and infantile function of language. (40)

In commenting briefly about how an adult, when pursuing thought

---

[8] Rubin, in his study, "The impact of the natural setting on private speech," (1979) concurs with Shields' finding that such private speech dialogues actually present the more advanced communication skills of young children, demonstrating non-egocentric role-taking and turn-taking skills (291).

on an inquiry, imagines himself speaking with his collaborators, Piaget does not explain this as a later development of imaginal dialogues in egocentric speech or symbolic play. Piaget does assign a positive function to this imaginal dialogue with the members of one's profession. He considers it a kind of rehearsal which assures that when one does actually speak to others about one's ideas they will already be "socially elaborated" and therefore roughly adapted to the audience. Thus imaginal dialogues in adulthood aid in the socializing of thought and in making one's communication of ideas better adapted to the reality of the listener. In his example, Piaget radically restricts both the imaginal audience (fellow professionals) and the circumstances which evoke such dialogue (pursuing an inquiry). But even without these restrictions, the functional significance Piaget attributes—the socialization of thought and the rehearsal of actual encounters—strengthens his commitment to an adaptationist point of view.

Piaget's vision of intelligence and conceptual thought narrows these to a set of formal logical operations not dependent on images. The model thinker for Piaget is the scientist or the logician, and not the artist, the dramatist, novelist, poet, or holy person. To the degree that the child's thought mirrors Piaget's image of the scientist's, the child is seen as possessing cognitive maturity.

Sutton-Smith (1911), a critic of Piaget's point of view, argues that while Piaget defines play as a function of cognition, he does not define the necessity or even the significance of play for cognition. From Piaget's perspective, Sutton-Smith asks, would adaptive thought be possible without symbolic play?

Vygotsky places monologal inner speech at the apex of verbal thought for three reasons: the functions he attributed to private speech and to verbal thought, his implicit conception of the self as unitary, and his consequent lack of focus on the presence of imaginal others in thought. Vygotsky's attribution of self-guidance and self-regulatory functions to private speech have shaped much of the contemporary research on such speech, as exemplified in a book edited by Zivin (1979). The research method employed by those sustaining the self-regulation paradigm has been for the most part to elicit speech by presenting the child with a cognitive task. It does indeed appear that speech during such occasions often has the function of planning and guiding behavior.

But this may be due to a circularity whereby the presupposed function of self-regulation dictates the research design and setting, which predictably produces examples of the kind of private speech favored by the theory. The reduction of all private speech to the function of self-regulation may therefore be an artifact of inquiries conducted within a restricted range of research contexts.

Shields' work on private speech opens a door out of this particular circularity by studying the private speech that occurs in imaginative play with objects. In the terrain of symbolic play such dialogues flourish. In Shields' observations the imaginal dialogues in the private speech of doll-play do not appear to show the increase in ellipsis that Vygotsky predicts with an increase in age. Rather the private speech in doll-play looks surprisingly like social speech. Shields does not observe in the imaginal dialogues of play the cognitive problem solving proposed by Vygotsky, or the inadequate attempts at communication proposed by Piaget. Her vignettes are dramatic in form. She sees their function as the creation of a world—much as Vygotsky sees the function of play.

Why wasn't Vygotsky interested in dialogues in egocentric speech and in inner speech? Let us propose that Vygotsky's focus on the function of self-regulation led him to data in which there was no clear articulation of characters and roles. When the child is focused on the execution of a task, the articulation of the imaginal process through which that is accomplished is absent. On the other hand, when the child has no goal in action to pursue (i.e, in play) the articulation of characters and scenes becomes more explicit.

To clarify this, let us consider an example from Kohlberg, Yaeger, and Hjertholm (1968). They present the following as an example of the self-guiding function of egocentric speech, calling it a "monologue description of one's own activity:"

> David (engaged in solitary play with a tinker toy, observer at desk at other side of room): The wheels go here, the wheels go here. Oh, we need to start it all over again. We need to close it up. See, it closes up. We're starting it all over again. Do you know why we wanted to do that? Because I needed it to go a different way. Isn't it going to be pretty clever, don't you think? But we have to cover up the motor just like a real car. (695)

In this "monologue" however, we find that the language is

dialogically structured with comment-acknowledgment, question-answer sequences. Further, the two "voices" have different functions or roles: one to put the tinker toy together, the other to facilitate this process, as a teacher might. In play, this dialogical structure might be made explicit through the use of puppets, one a child and one an older person. The child might be working on the tinker toy while the other tries to help, taking the role of a teacher.

> *David*: The wheels go here, the wheels go here. Oh, we need to start it all over again.
> *Teacher*: We need to close it up. See it closes up.
> *David*: We're starting it all over again.
> *Teacher*: Do you know why we wanted to do that?
> *David*: Because I needed it to go a different way. Isn't it going to be pretty clever, don't you think?
> *Teacher*: But we have to cover up the motor just like a real car.

If the primary agenda were completion of a task, however, such an explication of the dialogue would be unnecessary. It might even shift the focus from self-guidance of behavior and execution of the task to an imaginal conversation between two characters.

Vygotsky, like Piaget, did not allow his observations of imaginal dialogues in solitary play to influence his theory of the functions of private speech. Had Vygotsky allowed himself to be guided more by the phenomena of private speech in their multiplicity of appearances and less by his presumption of the centrality of the self-regulation function, perhaps the functions he attributed to play would have transformed his overall conception of private speech.

According to Vygotsky, play is used by the child to satisfy needs that reality cannot. In the imaginary situations which a child creates, unrealizable desires can be fulfilled (1978, 93). The ability to play is the power the child has to create another reality. This power is made possible by the ability of the child to subordinate action to meaning. Play releases the child from the dictatorship of the visual realm and the "incentive supplied by external things" and allows the child to act with meanings, to rely on internal tendencies and motives (96). Rather than stressing play's egocentrism, as Piaget does, Vygotsky is impressed with the fruits of such a liberation for a child's continued action in the social domain. In claiming that play is the highest level of preschool development, he attributes to play the propensity for creating voluntary intentions, to form real plans and volitional motives (103).

By defining inner speech as speech for oneself and external speech as for others, Vygotsky leaves no room for imaginal others—be they aspects of self, representations of known others, or wholly imaginary others. He assumes that the internal speaker knows what he or she is talking about and perceiving. There is no separate interlocutor or listener. But if we were to introduce a notion of the self as non-unitary, as having multiple points of view among which it alternates, dialogue would no longer be an inferior form of thought. Perhaps monologue would be appropriate in many instances. The degree of ellipsis (when present) might be understood as it is in speech (see E. Kaplan, 1952)—as reflecting the degree of intimacy among conversational partners. Vygotsky compares the degree of ellipsis in internal speech to that found in conversation between lovers, which he illustrates with a dialogue between Tolstoy's characters Kitty and Levin. But Vygotsky assumes that inner speech is elliptical not because the self is speaking with a character or figure it knows well, but because the only speaker is also the listener. Ellipsis in internal speech might also be due to the degree of intimacy among conversational partners.

Vygotsky argues that the monologue is superior to the dialogue (1962, 144), but to reach this conclusion he compares the monologue of thought to the dialogue of social speech. Can we assume that the latter is the same as the dialogue of internal speech? I think not. In the imaginal dialogues of thought, self and other do not necessarily share mutual perceptions. Thus when self and other are differentiated, one would expect internal speech to become less elliptical and more akin to spoken and written speech (the latter being, from Vygotsky's point of view, the most elaborate form of speech). In internal speech when self and a voice, or two voices, hold different perspectives, their views must be more fully elaborated than if one is entertaining and explicating a single view in a monologue. Through inner dialogue, a thought can be expressed by an imaginal other or by the self, questioned or furthered by another. Dialogue intensifies the way in which language carries us toward what we are going to understand, but as yet have not. "Thought germinates in speech" between others, says Merleau-Ponty, (1973, 131), and this is also true for the dialogues of thought. Before reasoning became synonymous with logical thought, its archaic meaning was "to engage in conversation or discussion" (Morris, 1969, 1036), as in *Isaiah* (1:18): "Come... Let us reason together." This conversation could have both actual and imaginal partners.

Turning next to Mead, we find that this understanding of reason is foundational to his psychology of thought. It is his notion of a development from the particularized imaginal others of children's play to the generalized other of adult thought that we wish to examine. In the nineteenth century—which Mead himself wrote about in fine detail—generalization was widely considered to be "necessary to the advancement of knowledge," but "particularity" was seen as "indispensable to the creatures of imagination" (Thomas Babington Macaulay 1825, quoted in Abrams, 1953, 316).

One anonymous nineteenth century writer, joining many of his contemporaries, equated science with:

> ...any collection of general propositions, expressing important facts concerning extensive classes of phenomena; and the more abstract the form of expression— the more purely it represents the general fact, to the total exclusion of such individual peculiarities as are not comprised in it—the more perfect the scientific language becomes.
>
> Science is the effort of reason to overcome the multiplicity of impressions, with which nature overwhelms it, by distributing them into classes, and by devising forms of expression which comprehend in one view an infinite variety of objects and events. (quoted in Abrams, 1953, 317)

Mead's emphasis on the generalized other clearly echoes these statements, affirming what might be described as a "scientific" form of thought rather than a poetic one. The generalized other is "the most inclusive or widest community included in one's organization of attitudes" (Miller, 1973, 49). In its highest development, says Mead, this would be analogous to a community of logicians.

The development of the generalized other is the development of socialized thought, wherein particular thoughts have the capacity to be conveyed to the widest possible audience. Such a generalization of imaginal others—a homogenization, it often sounds like—seems to be an important line of development. Its corollary, the fading out of the dramatic personae of thought, contradicts and obscures the development of particularized others, which "taken together, form a heterogeneous, accidental collection, a teething ring for utterances and not a ball team" (Goffman, 1981, 151).

Would it not make sense that these two developments—of particularized and generalized others—are not mutually contradictory but rather mutually dependent; that the generalized other does not always supplant particularized others, but that the form of the other (particularized or generalized) is dependent on the functions of the thought in a particular instance? If so, then for Mead to construct a developmental sequence from particularized to generalized other, his preferred *telos* must have again been scientific thought based on the model of nineteenth-century science. For Mead, imaginal others symbolize absent actual others where the imaginal is an internalization of social reality, whose purpose is adaptation to and preparation for social reality. When the imaginal is seen in this way, as merely a station between two moments of time in social reality, other functions of imaginal others are surely neglected.

CHAPTER FIVE

Imagination as Reality

What is meant by "reality?" It would seem to be something very erratic, very undependable—now to be found in a dusty road, now in a scrap of newspaper in the street, now in a daffodil in the sun. It lights up a group in a room and stamps some casual saying. It overwhelms one walking home beneath the stars and makes the silent world more real than the world of speech—and then there it is again in an omnibus in the uproar of Piccadilly. Sometimes, too, it seems to swell in shapes too far away for us to discern what their nature is.

—Virginia Woolf, 1929, 113-114

How different Woolf's vision of reality is from that of mechanistic philosophy's. Whitehead characterizes the latter as "a dull affair, soundless, scentless, colourless; merely the hurrying of material endlessly, meaninglessly" (1925, 56). In Woolf's vision, the real darts between the social world, the world of nature, and the world of things; it darts not alone but hand-in-hand with the imaginal.[9] How different from conceptions of the real as only the external and the material, of the imaginal as a confusion of wish-laden

---

[9] Hillman (1982) reminds us that in ancient Greek physiology, as in Biblical psychology, the heart was the organ for both sensation and imagination. Thus, sensing/perceiving the world and imagining the world were not conceived of separately, as they were later by the Scholastics, Cartesians, and British Empiricists. In these later psychologies sensing facts (inevitably about the external, material world) and intuiting fantasies are radically distinguished, sundering the connections between reality and imagination.

distortions! Certainly these views illumine some of our experience of the imaginal as a needed preserve against the harshness of reality. The word "real" functions not to tell what something is, but rather to delineate what it is not. It excludes possible ways of being "not real." The problem is that what "real" is cannot be pinned down in general, as it differs in various contexts. In dealings with imagining, the words "real" and "reality" are abused. Sarbin states:

> The traditional diagnostician uses these words in two ways: he says, for example, "the patient claims the hallucinated object has reality or is real;" that "the patient is out of contact with reality or the real world." The non-identity of the meaning of "real" for the diagnoser and the patient reflects some of the problems in the employment of the words real and reality. (1967, 376)

Different notions of the real yield vastly different valuations of imagining.

Let us therefore turn a corner and search out other perspectives on the real and see where they would lead imaginal dialogues and how they would understand the functions of these imaginal conversations. In doing so we shall turn to religion, aesthetics, and philosophy to put into question the presuppositions of those contemporary developmental theories which regard the imaginal as a distortion of reality, or as derivative from and subservient to external, material, and social reality.

We follow this course not because we tacitly subscribe to a religious ontology. Rather, we seek points of view which are different enough from developmental psychology's that the very contrast shall enable us to reflect more precisely on the nature of our usual theoretical commitments.

Imaginal Dialogues as Mirrors of Reality or Its Creator?

The contemporary Western psychological world view claims that images are internalizations of material and social reality which serve the function of representing this reality. In aesthetics this corresponds to the view that the mind and the imagination are reflectors of external objects—their mirrors—and that the function of art and of imagination is to reproduce external reality. From this perspective, the process of invention consists in "a reassembly of 'ideas' which are literally images, or replicas of sensations; and the resulting art work [is] itself comparable to a mirror presenting a selected and ordered image of life" (Abrams, 1953, 69). Divergences between the image and what it was modeled after—always a problem in such theories—are dealt with by mirror theorists in one of two ways. First, "any aesthetic apprehension which culminates in another view of objects and relations is viewed as a distortion or as a manifestation of pathology: at worst, a disease of the mind; a disease of the heart, at best" (Kaplan, 1981d, 7). Alternatively, art is seen as imitating not what we observe but what is "in" or "behind" what we observe, such as the Ideas or Forms which gave rise to nature as well as art (Abrams, 1953).

M. H. Abrams' book *The Mirror and the Lamp* (1953) contrasts this mimetic view with the expressive theory of art proposed by the Romantics. These theories are not presented as incompatible viewpoints to be chosen between, but as perspectives which allow us to see more of the complexity of the phenomenon of art. This is our own aim with respect to imaginal dialogues—not to pit one theory against another with the hope of one taking a last fall, but to see if we can begin to move more freely among viewpoints which have been banished from our developmental theorizing, as well as those sustained by our present conceptions.

In the Romantic view the imagination is not merely a replica of preexisting external reality. It has its own "internal source of motion;" it does not merely represent scenes but creates them (Abrams, 1953, 22, 25). When images of the natural or social world are evoked they do not function as copies of the "real," but rather serve to symbolize something else, often emotions[10] and experiences.

This is a radical shift. It demands a change in our developmental notions. Because a copy theory of perception views images as replicating the external world, then divergences between image and external referent are taken as pathognomic, as developmentally inferior to those images which faithfully copy natural or social reality. Thus we have arrived at theories stressing that development coincides with an increasing realism. But if the mind and the imagination

---

[10] "Not these plants, not these mountains, do I wish to copy, but my spirit, my mood, which governs me just at the moment..." said Tieck, a German Romantic (quoted in Abrams, 1953, 50).

are seen as contributing creatively to perception, then divergence between image and some external reality need not be negative. As soon as we allow that the image represents something other than the external, realism is no longer the measure, but rather the fit between the symbol and the symbolized. To achieve this fit, all manner of "distortions" of natural or social reality may be called for, and their achievement must be seen as a sign of development.

Etienne Gilson, discussing the painter Eugene Delacroix, wrote:

> But a true painter does not borrow his subject from reality; he does not even content himself with arranging the material provided by reality so as to make it acceptable to the eye. His starting point is fantasy, imagination, fiction, and all the elements of reality that do not agree with the creature imagined by the painter have to be ruthlessly eliminated. (1957, 130)

James Hillman discusses this conflict of possible interpretations in *Re-Visioning Psychology*, in which he describes the "naturalistic fallacy"—the tendency to judge "images to be right or wrong (positive or negative) largely by standards of naturalism. The more like nature an image appears, the more positive; the more distorted the image, the more negative" (1975b, 84). Taking issue with this approach, Hillman (1975b) argues:

> A multicolored child, a woman with an erected penis, an oak tree bearing cherries, a snake becoming a cat who talks, are neither wrong, false, nor abnormal because they are unnatural. Figures of the imagination are not restricted to jungles and zoos; they can crouch upon my bookshelf or stalk the corridors of last night's motel. (85-86)

A. C. Bradley, in his *Oxford Lectures on Poetry,* argues that poetry's nature is not to be

> a part, nor yet a copy, of the real world...but to be a world by itself, independent, complete, autonomous; and to possess it fully you must enter that world, conform to its laws, and ignore for a time the beliefs, aims and particular conditions which belong to you in the other world of reality...
>
> [Life and poetry] are parallel developments which nowhere meet, or, if I may use loosely a word which will be

serviceable later, they are analogous... They have different kinds of existence. (1920, 4, 6, 23-24)

Similarly, Elder Olson insists that poetic statements are not propositions, and "since they are not statements about things which exist outside the poem, it would be meaningless to evaluate them as true or false" (1942, 210-211).[11]

In the extreme the naturalistic fallacy operates not only to dictate the kinds of characters, the images of self and others which form imaginal dialogues, but to negate and discontinue the existence of such dialogues in thought and private speech. For instance for Vygotsky, when there is no actual interlocutor for whom our speech or thought is intended, our speech should not suggest that there is. If it does so anyway it is not yet efficient; it is insufficiently developed. Thought should reflect material reality. Dialogue that occurs in solitude is superfluous, at best. But what if thought is inherently dramatic and thus dialogical? Then, as Kaplan has said, it is the existence of monologues that we must account for!

Werner (1948) emphasizes the multiplicity of possible worlds and realities to a greater extent than the other developmental psychologists we have so far considered. He maintains that different kinds of creatures experience different "psychological worlds," and that within each of these psychological worlds there are various "spheres of reality." Pretend play and its imaginal dialogues are seen in this framework as symbolizing activity. "This paradigm," says Franklin, "takes as basic the idea that symbolizing does not—in its basic form—merely reflect or communicate what is already known but is formulative, meaning creating" (1981, 14).[12] Play creates a reality. From this point of view, development is not seen "as a linear (or spiralling) progression directed towards adaptation to a preexisting 'external reality' or (alternatively) towards the construction of a psychological reality dominated by a given mode of thought (such as the 'scientific')," but is a "differentiation, progressive construction and integration of spheres within psychological reality" (Franklin, 1981, 2-3). Observations

---

[11] Maritain (1953) sees this liberation from "realism" as at the same time a process of liberation from "conceptual, logical, discursive reason" (80). This is apparent in the work of the surrealists, for example, which follows neither the rules of realism nor of reason, but through improbable juxtapositions creates a new reality with its own set of meanings (Gilson, 1957).

[12] See Werner and Kaplan, 1963/1984; Kaplan 1981d.

of young children—Piaget's included—can be used to support the developmental notion that children are increasingly able to diverge in their imagery from a replication of material and social reality and not just that their images become more realistic.

Lowe (1975), in her study of the development of representational play in infants, maintains that at first the child applies his own activities (being fed, being combed, and being put to bed) to himself, and that with increasing age these are applied to the doll. So at first the doll is known through what the child does to it. The child makes the doll the object of activities that the child has previously been the object of. In so doing, the former object (the child) becomes the subject or agent (the one who performs the activities on another). This kind of play liberates children from the object role which so often characterizes the early dependence of the infant. It allows children to reflect from a distance upon the roles which are necessarily theirs.

At first the imaginal other is a passive recipient of the child's attention. Lowe suggests that it is not coincidental that the age at which the child begins to animate the doll is the same age at which the child begins to put words together (approximately 21 months). Indeed, she claims that some de-centering is necessary for both activities. She suggests that as a verbal component is added to these early action sequences, there is a "progressive animation of the doll, culminating at a point where the doll becomes an agent in its own right rather than a recipient of the child's care" (1975, 45).

Lowe notes that around 30 months of age, the children in her study would sometimes both express an awareness of their identification with the doll ("like the girl who placed the doll prone on its bed with the comment 'I sleep like that'") and would attribute their own dislikes to the doll ("She doesn't want to go to bed;" "She says she doesn't want dinner"). It would seem that with the acquisition of language the imaginal other can begin to be more than just a passive recipient of the imaginer's actions and it can begin to be articulated with respect to feelings and desires. However, this does not mean that the onset of language necessarily entails more animation and articulation of the other with respect to psychological properties. One finds even in the imaginal dialogues of adults that the other may be presented as a mere shadow or stick figure.

As the imaginal other is granted its own animation and agency, it can surprise the imaginer with its words. The imaginal other can act upon the self as well as be acted upon. Thus the range of situations which can be represented is enlarged, since one can now become the object of the other's actions just as the other was earlier the object of one's own actions.

If one analyzes the imaginal dialogues presented by Piaget in *Play, Dreams and Imitation* (1962b), the identity of the imaginal other appears to go from a vague younger child (i.e., the child's own role with respect to actual others), to the child's mother, to someone outside the child's family but known to the child, to someone heard about but not known, to a character which is entirely a creation of the child's mind. Both Piaget (1962b, 130) and Vygotsky (1978, 103) note how in the beginning the imaginary situations between self and imaginal other are repetitions or transmutations of the child's actual experiences. Only gradually does there ensue a shift from the simple "transposition of real life to the creation of imaginary beings for which no model can be found" (Piaget, 1962b, 130). Piaget observed play in which imaginary lands were created. The action in these worlds extended over time and involved increasingly complex scenarios and relations between characters. For instance Sachs' 10-year-old daughter complained to her mother that it was very "hard to use her model horses in play with new friends because they did not know the characteristics of each horse and the history of the herd" (Sachs, 1980).

The liberation of characters' identities from a narrow repertoire of known others is not only experienced in imaginal dialogues with respect to the role of the other, but even with respect to the role the child herself takes in these dialogues. Turning again to the protocols in *Play, Dreams and Imitation* (Piaget, 1962b), "J." is first herself, then either herself or a mothering-caretaking figure, and only five months later a person outside the mother-child dyad (i.e., the farmer's wife, and then the postman). Still later she plays the role of a real person whom she has never met before, only heard of. And finally, she is an imaginary being altogether. Piaget points out that only when his subjects reached two years of age was there a transition from attempting to imitate actions of the other while continuing to be oneself to actually becoming the other. Research carried out by Garvey (1979) and Garvey and Berndt (1977) has identified three stages the child passes through in becoming the other: 1) the child acts the role of the self in relation to the imaginal other; 2) during a transitional phase, the child neither is herself nor has she assumed a role; 3) the child takes on imaginal identities.

In psychoanalytic theory as well as in Piagetian theory, the movement from direct imitation to portrayal of imaginal others for whom no direct model can be ascertained is neutralized by a theory of distortion concerning imagery and the imagination. Just as the child's images begin to flower, the distortion theory explains, they must disguise themselves in order to elude the censorship of repression. So they are tidied up. Characters change role and costume. The characters of social reality—mother, father, brother—don the costumes of fancy. Through interpretation the make up is taken off, revealing once again the reals and knowns of Freud's reality. But a lion image which is interpreted to be a little boy's father may not simply be an instance of distortion, attempting to spare the boy the anxiety of dealing directly with the father image. If we turn to Jung, we find a different theory of symbolism that helps us escape from such total reduction to external reality. Here the character of the lion serves quite a different function, that of symbolizing an idea which is not yet known and whose best expression at the moment is this lion. In other words, the symbol does not reiterate what is already known but attempts to give form to what is not yet realized in its particularity. Kaplan calls this a "radical aesthetic," where "aesthetic creation is the imaginative realization of some lived-through, had experience, which would—save for the aesthetic activity—resist objectivity and realization" (1981d, 7). It is the "bringing of experiences and enjoyments out of the darkness of mere existence into the bright sunshine of contemplation and knowledge"; it is the "giving of significant form to what is otherwise 'unbodied,' formless" (Kaplan, 1981d, 7, 10).

To return to the image of the lion we need to study carefully the rest of the image's context. It is not evident simply from "lion" which attributes of lion are salient, which are hidden but meaningful, and which are inappropriate. A lion may scare its accompanying partner, but this frightening aspect may actually be less meaningful than the respect the lion commands in his terrain. Although these characteristics are indeed inextricable, they can be arranged in different hierarchies of meaning. The lion may very well have reference to the father. But as we pay closer attention to the image of the lion, its meaning goes beyond simple synonymy with the father. As we all know, the child encounters many lion-like aspects in the world.

Such symbolization of course pertains to the role of the self as well. Role taking is often seen as the child's attempt to assimilate societal roles other than his own, and their perspectives on himself. However, with symbolization in mind the child never just practices a role but uses the role as well to express himself and to create an alternative world. Thus one is not a policeman for the mere practice function of exploring "policeman" as a role, but because issues of power, protection, and vulnerability are afoot. To look at it in this way is similar to dream interpretation where one must ask, "Why out of all the possible day residues, is it this particular detail around which a dream has grown?" The child does not ask himself how to express a sense of some naughtiness. He becomes and acts the part of a dirty, slippery, hungry little pig. Instead of saying one is needy, one acts the part of a crying, hungry, whining infant. This enacting is not only relevant to understanding children and adults' dreams and imaginal dialogues, but also to changes of tone and voice in conversation.

This line of development, away from images as imitations of reality to images as creators of new worlds has been overshadowed by Piaget's and Vygotsky's assumption that this form of play gradually fades as games with rules replace it. Rather than join the debate over whether play is exclusively replication, reconstruction, or transformation, Franklin (1981) offers the alternative of delineating two tendencies in pretend play (and, I would add, in imaginal dialogues): one toward realism, the other toward the fantastical. While the fantastical by definition breaks the rules of everyday reality, there is within such play a development toward greater inner coherence, just as in reality-oriented play. Such movement toward inner coherence, Franklin remarks, characterizes all forms of world-making. In imaginal dialogues this might mean that characterizations of self and others become more stable, that dialogues follow the rules of conversation, or that individual situations begin to coalesce into more structured and well-defined worlds of particularized relations.

This differentiation between realistic and fantastical development of images and imaginal dialogues is an old one. The notion that imaginal dialogues are copies or imitations of actually occurring dialogues is of course suggested in the very root of the term imagination—

imago, an imitation or copy. If we turn to Vico, we find him differentiating between *imaginatio* and *phantasia*. In the latter one does not simply represent the given (as in the former), but creates or brings something new into being. Thus, the image is liberated from a position of inferiority with respect to external reality, as "image does not represent a given. It is a given...[it] is not an extension of reality. It is the novelty in the sense of creating something new from a present reality... It is the making of reality itself" (Verene, 1979, 47-48).

Recent research has also helped to dispel the prejudiced conception that involvement with imaginal companions necessarily conflicts with involvement in reality and with interpersonal relations—and is thus suggestive of pathology. Singer in 1973 studied 141 three- and four-year olds, and found that 65 percent reported having imaginary playmates. The children who reported having such companions were less aggressive, more cooperative, smiled more, were better able to concentrate, were less frequently bored, and were more linguistically advanced than their companionless cohorts. They were clearly cognizant of the difference between external reality and the worlds of their imagination. There was no indication that these children as a group were supplanting object relations with fantasy.[13] Similarly a study done in 1968 by Lewinsohn of patients with hallucinations found that other psychiatric patients judged the hallucinating ones to be more friendly and less defensive and to have more positive expectations regarding others than non-hallucinating patients.

Personifying

The intelligible forms of ancient poets
the fair humanities of old religion...
...all these have vanished.
They live no longer in the faith of reason!
But still the heart doth need a language, still
Doth the old instinct bring back old names...

—Coleridge's expanded translation of part of
Schiller's "Die Piccolomini"

---

[13] Hillman (1977) and Watkins (1981a) also note that in psychotherapeutic work with adults, imaginal figures often desire not to separate their fleshly conversant from daily life, but to be taken by the imaginer into the world. See the case presented in Chapter Twelve in this regard.

IMAGINATION AS REALITY

For the Romantics the poet's creation of imaginary beings, the personification of virtues, vices, passions and nature, likened the poet to God, joining Him in the peopling of worlds, in bringing "possibility over into the realm of being" (Abrams, 1953, 288).[14] The poet and the painter may use the natural world, but their intention is to create with it a new world, another world—which has been called a "heterocosm" (Abrams, 1953, 27).[15] At the center of this other world, this alternate world, are imaginal others. We hear this in the words of Romantics such as Addison, Young, Aiken, Warton.

> [Poetry] has not only the whole circle of nature for its province, but makes new worlds of its own, [and] shews us persons who are not to be found in being… (Addison, quoted in Abrams, 1953, 275)

For Young the human mind "in the vast void beyond real existence…can call forth shadowy beings, and unknown worlds." And in John Aiken's mind, the imagination could not be content with "the bounds of natural vision," and quickly "peoples the world with new beings…embodies abstract ideas" (both quoted in Abrams, 1953, 382).

For Joseph Warton, writing in 1753, personification is the peculiar privilege of poetry and ingredient to a lively imagination:

> It is the peculiar privilege of poetry…to give Life and motion to immaterial beings; and form, and colour, and action, even to abstract ideas; to embody the Virtues, and Vices, and the Passions… Prosopopoeia, therefore, or personification, conducted with dignity and propriety, may be justly esteemed one of the greatest efforts of the creative power of a warm and lively imagination (quoted in Abrams, 1953, 289)

Whereas developmental and psychoanalytic psychologies focus on how the imaginal other is an internalization of actual others, or of aspects

---

[14] W. B. Yeats, in speaking of elves, spirits, fairies, and goblins said, "all nature is full of invisible people…some of these are ugly or grotesque, some wicked or foolish, many beautiful beyond any one we have ever seen, and…the beautiful are not far away when we are walking in pleasant and quiet places" (Arrowsmith and Moorse, 1977).

[15] In a discussion of the painter Delacroix, Gilson (1957) said that "the final casue of all operations performed by a pianter is to casue the existence of a self-subsisting and autonomous being—namely the particular painting freely concieved by his imagination" (131).

of them—albeit often disguised and distorted representations—the Romantics and others see imaginal beings as donning the costumes of figures in the upper world. Personifying is not an anachronistic relic of social life which serves merely to compensate for absent or inadequate "real" people. The personifications in dreams and imaginal dialogues are not always or only by-products of "schizoid operations"— "a splitting of the ego in the service of defense, with a consonant splitting of a fundamental, core object that was libidinally invested and yet frustrating at the same time" (Kernberg, 1980, 61). From the Romantic point of view personifying, which occurs naturally in dreams, myth, poetry, and play, is a process which underlies thinking and is reflective of the poetic nature of the mind. It is not merely that the mind can conjure up figures to represent abstract ideas, but that Virtue, Evil and their respective hordes appear as persons.

Thus Hillman defines personifying as "the spontaneous experiencing, envisioning and speaking of the configurations of existence as psychic presences" (1975b, 12), and differentiates it from personification, animism, and anthropomorphism. Animism and anthropomorphism imply that the imaginer has made certain category errors by either attributing living soul to inanimate objects or by projecting human attributes to inhuman forms. With the term personification, the emphasis is on the self's attribution of its own characteristics to a thing or abstraction.

Wordsworth criticized earlier poets such as Dryden, Gray, and Cowper for using personifying as a rhetorical device, and thereby denying its religious dimension. For Coleridge and Wordsworth, personification, as animism and symbolism, were "to move and please the reader" and were "natural expressions of the 'creative imagination'" (Abrams, 1953, 292). These imaginal others were not moved as puppets, but were experienced as autonomously affecting their listener. Recently Wordsworth's criticism has been resumed in the writings of Jung and Hillman. Both stress that imaginal others appear not just through conscious attempts to personify, but are experienced at times as being outside of and independent of one's conscious agency. In their treatment of imaginal others there is no pressure for experience to conform to a theory of projection (i. e., for such others to be eventually experienced as self or as created by self.) Instead it is emphasized that the experience of self changes through dialogue with an imaginal other. It seems as though the imaginal other is creating the self, as much as the self is creating the imaginal other. These imaginal persons bring us up as surely as our parents, not simply as substitutes for our parents, but as companions in imaginal worlds. And it is not only children who invite imaginal others to the dinner table. Machiavelli had imaginary dinner conversations with historical personages (Hillman, 1975b, 199). Petrarch wrote letters to the eminences of classical antiquity. Landor (1915) wrote volumes of imaginal dialogues between sages and stars of different centuries. Pablo Casals (1967) told his listeners, "Bach is my best friend." It seems art, drama, poetry, music, as well as the spontaneous appearance of personifications, keep us in conversation with imaginal others. From this point of view these imaginal others affect our interactions with "actual" others just as surely as the other way around.

Whereas psychoanalysis has tried to cope with the differences between actual and imaginal others by saying the imaginal is a representative of an external reality, other psychological theorists such as Jung and Melanie Klein have taken other routes. Each noticed that imaginal others and their scenarios cannot be accounted for even by a detailed examination of the person's experience in the social and external world. For each it was necessary to posit some other factor apart from internalization to explain the deviations between the real and the imaginal. For Jung, this was accomplished by his notion of archetypes: one inherits forms through which one experiences. The form is distinct from and prior to experience, although dependent on experience for its expression as a particular image. Due to Klein's emphasis on biology, her puzzlement at the discrepancy between children's imaginal family figures and their actual parents was put to rest by a theory of instinct. In her model the powerful life and death instincts reshape experience to formulate the character of particular imaginal others and their scenes.

Both of these theorists introduce a factor, logically prior to experience in the external world, which attempts to account for the fact that imaginal others are not always representations of "actual" others. In each theory, as in Romantic notions of mind, the mind does not just passively receive external images but has a role in actively constructing "what is done with what is seen" (Abrams, 1953, 57). For Klein this constructive capacity of mind pointed to biological substrata.

For Jung, it pointed toward the universals of myth, religion and art. The basic similarity of these moves, despite their apparent difference, is suggested by one of Klein's students, W. R. Bion. While Klein advanced the postulate that children have an innate knowledge of the genitals of both sexes and of sexual intercourse, Bion (1962, 1963) elaborated this by "postulating an innate preconception of the Oedipus myth" (Kemberg, 1980, 41).

In all three cases—Klein, Jung, Bion—one is struck by a similarity of intuition: fantasies cannot be understood solely with reference to a process of internalization, that the contents of fantasy go beyond the child's experience, and that they do so in ways that can be classified by the observer into certain common patterns or structures. The problem of how fantasy and its persons can go beyond experiences in the social realm is usually approached by way of some innate contribution, and this usually leads to some mythical conception: a death instinct, archetypes, innate myths. The final conceptualization often obscures the validity of the initial observation, namely, that there is a limit to what the processes of internalization and the mechanisms of defense can account for in the life of the imaginal.

This does not mean to underestimate the contributions of our psychoanalytic understandings of defense and internalization. These have provided the theory and technique that guide the daily practice of psychotherapy. Nor, in suggesting that development does not always coincide with an increasing realism, do we deny the fact that this is often the case. Let us agree for now with the object relations theorists in their insistence that there is a development from polarized ("black or white") figures to more complexly drawn, multidimensional figures. But, whereas their argument rests on imaginal figures replicating the complexity of actual human beings, our agreement will rest on how added complexity increases the power, autonomy, and differentiation of the imaginal as symbolic in Jung's sense. This increasing complexity in characterization need not necessarily balance out good and bad qualities. In the imaginal, evil and good figures can exist in great complexity of delineation. There is still room for the Queen of the Night, for Mephistopheles, and the Virgin Mary.

If personification is seen as an aspect of mind which arises naturally rather than only as a result of schizoid operations, then multiplicity of figures is viewed differently. For Fairbairn the ego is at first unitary and pristine, then under environmental stress it splits into various voices. This becomes exacerbated in schizoid conditions. Thus positive development is equated with a reduction of this splitting of the endopsychic structures. Adding more characters would seem to be negative. In this model multiplicity is the result of a pathognomic process resulting in representations that are one-sided and superficial. But what if the birth of a new character (or set of new characters!) was seen not as serving a defensive function, but one of symbolic representation? What if multiplicity of characters was not conceived of as synonymous with shallowness of character? Even if personification does first occur as a process of defense, as a reaction to external reality and its frustrations, need it continue to serve only as this? When personifying is construed positively as a symbolic event, then development does not coincide with a shift from multiplicity to integration into one, but with awareness of multiplicity.

Given psychoanalysis' original concern with pathology and its commitment to the priority of the external and the material, focus on the imaginal has most often involved a set of concerns about differentiating "pathological" from non-pathological phenomena: hallucination from perception, a concrete understanding of images from a metaphorical one, "unrealistic" representations from realistic ones. From the psychoanalytic perspective, imaginal life results from internalization of the external world and this process is itself seen in a pathological light, as we have described. This eye for pathology which derogates the products of internalization contrasts sharply with Mead's positive construal of the creation of the self and its internal world through internalization. To use psychoanalytic concepts to study imaginal dialogues thus implicitly reduces the phenomenon to concern with pathology. Reality testing becomes the pivotal activity.

For Freud psychical reality, the reality of the imagination, was both derivative from and subordinate to external reality. It had no truly independent status as a reality. If we see some imaginal dialogues as creative—which does not rule out their having borrowed elements from actual conversations and people—then we are confronted with various modes of the real which may be hierarchically organized in different ways depending on the preferred goal in a specific situation.

Casey argues that Freud's conception of reality was too narrow to include the richness of his own observations about psychical reality.

He proposes that a more adequate model would acknowledge the validity of two different types or modes of reality: objective and experiential. "Objective reality" would denote that:

> ...realm of definite entities—material, social, or even psychological—regarded as potential objects of scientific knowledge. The objectively real would be that towards which a consensus of impartial inquirers tends. In Peirce's model, these inquiries "converge" on the objectively real without always, or perhaps ever, attaining it as such. This kind of reality is not always or necessarily experienced) it may possess only posited or constructed status without losing its objectivity. In any case, the idea of objective reality allows both for Freud's concern for scientific objectivity and for his skepticism with regard to the ultimate knowability of the real. (Casey, 1971-72, 684)

While realism may be the developmental measure for objective reality, it is not always for experiential reality. The mother figure who rapes the dreamer in a dream or waking dream could be entirely at odds with objective reality, and yet capture an experiential reality in a most apt and poignant way. As Casey points out, the shift from objective to experiential reality entails a shift in the nature of representations from being indicative to being expressive (1971-72, 687).

The Real as Inclusive of the Imaginal

When imagination is seen purely as a substitute for a deficient external reality, then it is derogated for its wishing. Wishing is seen as a childish affair that intervenes in the attempt to adapt to reality. It is a sign of inability or unwillingness to make peace with "what is," with what is real. When imagination is seen as creative of realities, wish is construed positively as a longing that gives rise to this creation. From this point of view imaginal dialogues do not merely ameliorate a harsh reality but are active in the construction of imaginal realities.

An illustration of this creation of other realities through wish and longing and the imaginal dialogues that result is given in Corbin's (1969, 1980) treatment of Ibn 'Arabi and Avicenna, mystics of the tenth and eleventh centuries. The relevance of Corbin's studies, as documents of psychology and not just of history of religions, is that he sought not to present Avicenna *per se*, but the Avicennean experi-

IMAGINATION AS REALITY

ence. He is interested in the "mode of perception" and of being implicit in Avicenna's work (Corbin, 1980, 8). In the Persian mysticism of Ibn 'Arabi and Avicenna, imaginal dialogues between men and their angels form the central experience around which a cosmology of levels and worlds revolves. One comes to know oneself through coming to know one's Lord, one's Angel. Each person and Angel comes into being through the other, not all at once, but gradually through being with each other. In Ibn 'Arabi's words,

> We have given Him to manifest Himself through us, whereas He has given us (to exist through Him). Thus the role is shared between Him and us... If He has given us life and existence by His being, I also give Him life by knowing Him in my heart.

The voice of his Angel said to him,

> If then you perceive me, you perceive yourself. But you cannot perceive me through yourself. It is through my eyes that you see me and see yourself, Through your eyes you cannot see me. (From Ibn 'Arabi's *Book of Theophanies*, quoted in Corbin, 1969, 127, 114)

For Ibn 'Arabi, to return to one's Lord is to "return to his self" "to *yourself* as you are known by your Lord" (Corbin 1969, 253). In "prayer there is between God and his faithful not so much a sharing of roles as a situation in which each by turns takes the role of the other" (264). Prayer is "a dialogue in which the two parties continually exchange roles" (269).

Were it not that Ibn 'Arabi's and Avicenna's interlocutors were Angels or Lords—were their interlocutors reduced to representations of "actual" others—we might hear echoes of G.H. Mead in these thoughts. For did not Mead believe that the Self is created through the child's transit into others' perspectives on him? Of course many in Mead's time argued that his system was implicitly religious, that the "generalized other" was not simply an amalgamation of the society's points of view, but represented God. Of this Mead could not be convinced. The opposing interpretations of course issued from conflicting ontological commitments: the secular and the non-secular.

In the systems of belief which Corbin presents, imaginal dialogue is prayer. Prayer is not a request for something, it is "a means of existing and of causing to exist, that is, a means of causing the God who reveals Himself to appear, of 'seeing' Him." He is seen not as He is, "in His essence," but in "the form" which this person's being or consciousness calls out. Thus the God does not exist in and of Himself with fixed qualities, but exists through dialogue with a particular man. "No theophany is possible except in the form corresponding to the predisposition of the subject" who receives the theophany (Corbin, 1969, 270).

In the psychological models we have been treating, the others of the everyday material world are given primacy. Imaginal others are derived. In many religious systems, God is primary and creates people. In Ibn 'Arabi's system man and God co-create each other. It is longing that begins prayer—both God's prayer to see Himself in a mirror which sees Him and man's prayer to become such a mirror (Corbin, 1969, 261). When one does not yet see one's Lord in his heart, he is urged to pray as though he saw Him, and in so doing to create the situation of longing in which the Angel appears.[16]

In the Avicennean and Suhrawardian recitals translated by Corbin, the development of the relation to the Angels is recounted, beginning with exodus from the material world, to an encounter with the Angel and the Angel's world (1980, 32). These recitals record the dialogues between person and imaginal interlocutor. The world of the Angels and the events that transpire there are symbolic in the sense earlier discussed: "the symbol is not an artificially constructed 'sign'"; it announces "something that cannot be expressed otherwise; it is the unique expression of the thing symbolized" (Corbin, 1980, 30). When the attention returns to events in the everyday world, this symbolic awareness raises everyday events to the level of the dream. This is, of course, the same direction of thought taken in the Italian Renaissance by people such as Ficino. Instead of seeing an opposition between the imaginal and the real, an analogical mode was suggested in which the real is viewed as imaginal and the imaginal as real, reality as a dream and dream as reality. For Ficino the world is thus a theater (Cope, 1973, 77). For Novalis, "the World becomes the Dream, the

---

[16] A Contemporary author, Marilynne Robinson, puts it this way in her novel *Housekeeping* (1980, 152-153): "For to wish for a hand on one's hair is all but to feel it. So whatever we may lose, very craving gives it back to us again. Though we dream and hardly know it, longing, like an angel fosters us, smooths our hair, and brings us wild strawberries."

IMAGINATION AS REALITY

Dream the World" (quoted in Cope, 1973).

Instead of the real and the imaginal being opposed as the imaginal distorts, condenses, rearranges and negates the real, it is thought that through the imaginal the truer nature of the real is manifested. It is the intermediate universe—the universe between pure spirit and the physical, sensible world—which is the world of the symbol and of imagining. In it spirits become corporealized and bodies spiritualized. This intermediate world, 'alam al mithal, the "*mundus imaginalis*," "corresponds to a precise mode of perception" which is imaginative power or perception (Corbin, 1972, 1). Corbin reflects his authors' intentions by arguing that this mode of perception, though not sense perception or intellectual intuition, is nonetheless every bit as real, or even more real. In this mode of perception development is not attendant to de-personification, to pure logic or abstract thought, to assimilating the imaginal other into the self, or forsaking him in loyalty to objective reality. Development has to do rather with attaining a state of mind, through longing, in which personifying occurs spontaneously. The resulting figures are not considered "imaginary" but "imaginal," in order to indicate that they are not unreal. For Corbin these imaginal others are part of the real, where the real is defined more largely than our modern Western conception of it. Dialogues with the "Angels" of imaginal reality, far from being symptomatic of pathology, are understood as teaching one to hear the events of the everyday symbolically and metaphorically.

The relevance of these ideas to our own psychology is best expressed by Corbin himself:

> Let us not make any mistake and simply state that our precursors in the West conceived imagination too rationalistically and too intellectualistically. Unless we have access to a cosmology structured similarly to that of the traditional Oriental philosophers, with a plurality of universes arranged in ascending order, our imagination will remain out of focus, and its recurrent conjunctions with our will to power will be a never-ending source of horrors. In that event, we would be confining ourselves to looking for a new discipline of the Imagination. It would, however, be difficult to find such a new discipline, as long as we continue to see in it no more than a way of getting a certain distance to what is called reality and a way of act-

ing upon reality. Now, this reality we feel is arbitrarily limited as soon as we compare it to the reality described by our traditional theosophers, and this limitation degrades reality itself. (1972, 16)

It is beyond the scope of this book to describe how the historical pressures of Christianity and the rise of science narrowed the prevailing conception of reality to exclude imaginal figures. Let it suffice to say that as long as reality is defined this narrowly, imaginal dialogues will be seen as either a means to adapt to that delimited reality or as a nuisance thwarting the desired adaptation—and our view of other possible functions of the imaginal will be distorted. From this constricted view of reality such dialogues become merely one among other ways to rehearse future social discourse, practice language skills, guide behavior. In psychotherapy this view results in such practices as teaching schizophrenics and hyperactive children to talk to themselves to guide their feelings and behavior and to adapt to the demands of external social reality. (See Meichenbaum, 1977 and Meichenbaum and Goodman, 1979.)

Once we open up reality to include the poetic, the dramatic, and the spiritual, the development of our relations with imaginal figures can no longer be confined to our customary notions. Development itself needs to be reconceived. Adaptation to reality changes its meaning, as reality becomes not just the sensible, material, and external reality, but created and imaginal realities as well. Adaptation with regard to a redefined notion of reality would no longer reflect a primarily "utilitarian, 'survival'—or 'achievement' oriented context" (Herron and Sutton-Smith, 1971, 2), but would include forming a relation to symbolic and expressive modes of thought. Sutton-Smith argues this point of view with respect to symbolic play, which is among the first sites of imaginal dialogues. Play, he argues, is not solely a cognitive (nor affective or conative) function but "an expressive form *sui generis* with its own unique purpose" (Sutton-Smith, 1971, 341). "Reverie and creative imagination have to do," he says, "with more novel forms of adaptation" (331). They are creative of realities and not just deficient ones expressive of the child's inability to accommodate himself to external reality or failure to relinquish a position of egocentricity. They are creative of alternate realities, of symbolic and metaphorical realities.

Corbin is not presented here to advocate a religious point of view with regard to imaginal dialogues. The virtue of the system he describes is that it begins with the experience of the imaginal other and illustrates how, when this experience is engaged, there can develop a metaphorical way of thinking, a reflection between mundane and imaginal realities that enriches them both. The developmental theories dealt with earlier approach imaginal dialogues from a theory of projection which too quickly moves from the experience of the figures to explanatory principles. If one lingers with the experience of the figures' autonomy, as Corbin's poets did, development is seen in terms of the manner of relating to the figures, rather than the gradual reabsorption and disappearance of the figures suggested by the psychological theories we have discussed.

CHAPTER SIX

The Impact of Conceptions of Development on Approaching Imaginal Dialogues

It is not a question here of how we must turn, twist, limit or curtail the phenomenon so that it can still be explained, if need be, by principles which we once agreed not to exceed, but it is a question rather of the direction in which we must expand our ideas to come to terms with the phenomenon.
 —Schelling, 1857 (quoted in Otto, 1981, 46)

Thus far we have been speaking of developmental approaches to imaginal dialogues without directly focusing on how the conceptions of development implicit in the theories presented have impacted the phenomenon under discussion. The critique of these developmental conceptions comes mainly from the organismic-developmental model.

Disentangling Development from Ontogenesis and Chronology

All of the developmental theories presented in Part I discuss the development of imaginal dialogues from an ontogenetic point of view. In other words, they discuss the emergence of and changes in such dialogues in private speech and thought from early childhood onwards. As Kaplan (1974) points out, many of our contemporary developmental theories, like evolutionary theories before them, fuse the idea of development with history and biography, such that temporally earlier forms are interpreted as relatively imperfect—destined to be extinguished, displaced by, or transformed into later, presumably higher, more perfect forms. Thus we see imaginal dialogues in play replaced by abstract thought, or those in private speech transmuted into the monologues of thought. For instance, the early display of imaginal dialogues in the symbolic play of childhood is ignored as possible evidence for the centrality and persistence of imaginal dialogues throughout life, or for the sophisticated ability of the preschooler to de-center, to speak for the imaginal other, to symbolize, to meet the rules of dialogal speech. Rather it is almost radically interpreted as something which is and ought to be lodged in childhood. Insofar as it appears in later life it is taken as persistence of primitivity. Much of developmental theory is constructed such that, except in cases of pathology, what is conceived of as "good" is evidenced in adulthood, and what is thought to be inferior is found in childhood and hopefully abandoned there. So too with our evaluations of ways of thinking in the earlier "childhood" of cultures before ours.

If this form of theorizing were not so prevalent, the child might indeed be "father of the man" with regard to imagination, as Blake suggested. What the analyst must infer about "self- and object-representations," from the adult patient's thoughts, feelings and interpersonal relations, the child spontaneously enacts in play—revealing the dramatic structure of psyche. What a curious state of affairs we have created when child analysts consistently refer the plethora of characters arising from play back to the self and the actual others of the child's daily life, while the adult analyst listens for the characters, the self- and object-representations, in the patient's talk of self and others! Were the adult not to relinquish the child's ability to "hear voices," then he and the analyst would be spared the task of making such inferences about the underlying imaginal structures of personality and perception.

*Development Concerns Not Simply What Is
But What Should Be*

The conflation of development with time encourages the misconception that developmental theorists simply observe what children do over time and report these "facts," adding to their inventory of skills the child's achievements through time. These "facts" are of course usually organized into some set of stages which are supposed to unfold over time, delivering a more perfect, more highly developed person (namely, the adult). Of course, this misconception serves to make developmental psychology akin to natural science. But development cannot simply be read from the "facts" of growing up. It is a perspective through which observations can be ordered.

> Development is a norm or standard for interpreting and assessing actualities, and cannot itself be derived from empirical observations or experimental analyses. (Kaplan, 1981b, 8)

The "facts" which theories claim are to be found in reality are, from this perspective, produced by the given theory. Different theories produce different sets of facts, depending on the views of the nature of mind and reality that inform them. The degree to which it appears that children do go through the stages outlined in a particular theory may be seen not as a sign of the unfolding of some natural process of development, but rather as a reflection of the extent to which children have been enculturated to share the goals of that theory and the culture that created it (see Toulmin, 1981, 261). There are limits to this viewpoint, including obvious exceptions such as the development of rudimentary motor skills or physiological development in general. Beyond this rudimentary level of development, however, we find that values organize the preferred *telos*.

Kaplan proposes that development be seen as a movement toward perfection. A developmentalist's task then is to describe not simply what is, but what should be (1981b, 5). When one looks in this way at theories of development, one sees what the given theorist specifies implicitly or explicitly as the primary goal, and how phenomena are then selectively gathered or discarded based on their ability to explain the primary problem. For instance for Piaget this "selection pressure led to a narrowing of the range of phenomena to those that seem most capable of relating to the development of logically necessary judgments...as the problem of logical form was taken as primary" (Glick, 1981, 11-12).

Formal Similarities

The ontogenetic approach toward imaginal dialogues has introduced confusion into what might otherwise have seemed straightforward. For instance, Piaget argues that symbolic play (and we should add its imaginal dialogues) is replaced by rule-governed games. Such games do indeed follow the early proliferation of imaginal scenes enacted by the child, and were symbolic play to be transmuted into such games, Piaget's thesis of a movement toward increasingly abstract and logic-oriented thought would be bolstered.

However, if we leave time as a measure of relation between two phenomena, we can focus on the degree of formal similarity instead. This focus allows us to see a clear relation between such things as the child's imaginal dialogues in play, adult fantasy, playwriting, and praying. In all of these there are two or more roles or characters, a scene and dialogue which function to create a world—fantastical, representative, or some mixture of the two. Instead of linking imaginal dialogues in the early play of children to logical thought, would not common sense have us see them as related to dialogues in dramas and novels, to authors' and poets' (and eventually readers') experiences of speaking with characters, to the imaginal dialogues of fantasy which suffuse adult thought, to adults' experience of dialogue with God or with aspects of nature? If we can agree on this, then it should be clear that development in these realms can not be defined by the achievement of a process of de-personification of the characters or by an integration of the multiplicity of characters into a single one. These two moves would dissolve the dramatic nature of these; dialogues and make it impossible for there to be dialogue at all! How would we go about saying what development would be?

The Preferred Telos of a Phenomenon Specifies What Constitutes Development

The level of development of a phenomenon cannot be assessed without taking into account the particular context of the phenomenon at a given time and the given *telos* or goal:

> ...there is no single "developmental course" or "sequence" in an individual's life. With different *teloi*, the relevant developmental "sequence" will be different. (Kaplan, 1981b, 17)

A phenomenon, such as speaking with an imaginal figure or primary process thought, therefore, would never be primitive *per se*. Most psychoanalytic discussions assume that "the primary processes and secondary processes are mutually antagonistic and that the former have, in health, to be relegated by repression to a curious underworld" (Rycroft, 1979, 158). But the kinds of thinking Freud claimed were characteristic of dream speech—distortion, condensation, displacement, over-determination—are not just "inferior kinds of thinking (looked at from the naturalistic viewpoint) but ways of speaking poetically, rhetorically, and symbolically" (Hillman, 1975b, 85). To judge whether an imaginal figure accurately represents someone "in reality" may miss the crucial distinction between the goal of representation of and the goal of representation as (Kaplan, 1981a, 23). This confusion has led many object relations therapists to use the kind of figures in dreams and fantasies to indicate level of object representation, rather than reading them as expressive of the psychological reality of the patient (see Watkins, 1978). For instance, a woman's dream of an imaginal figure, a haggard husband whose body is a wooden barrel, with glass chips pressed into the wood might be taken as evidence of the patient's inability to differentiate the inanimate and the animate—despite her proven ability to do so in her capacity to relate the dream in words to a human therapist, and regardless of (perhaps) the high degree of fit between the symbol and the symbolized.

Let us illustrate further how altering the *telos* changes the assessment of the phenomenon. For Piaget the high degree of assimilation in symbolic play contributed to his pejorative assessment of it. This of course would be required if the primary developmental goal were accommodation and adaptation to the demands of external reality. But for poet William Blake assimilation was not just tolerated but given the highest value. A high degree of assimilation was not egocentric, because by first assimilating the world into oneself, one could create other worlds (Engell, 1981, 248). The creation of imaginal worlds was the primary goal. Whereas Piaget saw play as egocentric, the Romantics (and Mead as well) would have seen its imaginal dialogues as instrumental to the development of "sympathy." That is, through such dialogues the child, like the poet,

> may be said, for the time, to identify himself with the character he wishes to represent, and to pass from one to

another, like the same soul successively animating different bodies. (William Hazlitt, quoted in Abrams, 1953, 245)

The imagination, far from being a domain of self-centered wishes, was for Shelley and others the organ by which the individual could exercise sympathy, understanding, and moral goodness by identifying himself with others.

The multiplicity of developmental courses suggested in the literature concerning imaginal dialogues results from theorists' advocating different *teloi* as primary: the development of abstract thought, of social discourse, or of adaptation to reality. These different *teloi*, of course, would lead one to select different series of changes during childhood to focus on. For instance, the child first knows the imaginal other (the doll, the imaginary companion) through her own activities. The imaginal other is at first a passive recipient of the child's attention and action. Only gradually does the doll become animated and act as an agent in its own right. Also at first, the doll is used to represent either the child herself or people the child knows intimately—brother, sister, mother, father. Then there is a shift to people the child knows less well (mailman, teacher), then to people the child has heard of but never met, and finally to totally imaginary beings. Thus characters are gradually released from being props to the ego's actions and pale reflections of the already known. As characters become animated and autonomous it is possible to find out about the details of their relationships and their world, not just how they impinge on the self.

If we follow these lines of development we find ourselves rehearsing not for Piaget's scientific audience, not for actual social discourse, and not for action or a harsh reality, but rather, as Hillman has said, we find ourselves rehearsing for imaginal life itself—that other life where we are also housed, clothed, and cared for. That other life of dialogue also creeps into our gestures, our turns of phrase, the very structure of our thought, just as surely as it presents itself in our dreams and waking dreams, in art and poetry, novels and prayer. Robert Kiely points out in his discussion of Virginia Woolf that:

> ...through the imagination, the individual can escape exile and confinement and dwell momentarily with shepherds and queens. But the exercise of imagination involves more than inventing situations and characters, it is...a movement of mind and heart from one vantage point to

another. It is not merely a multiplication of flat scenes, but an entrance into the dimensionality of experience beyond the self, a leap from the balcony to the stage, from silence to speech. (1980, 223)

Imaginal dialogues can be a means of creating worlds, of developing imaginative sympathy through which we go beyond the limits of our own corporeality and range of life experiences by embodying in imagination the perspectives of others, actual and imaginal. Through this relating to imaginal others (whether they be created by a novelist, by the self, or whether they arise spontaneously) our own habitual point of view (often called the ego's) may be relativized and placed in relation to those of others. Virginia Woolf speaks of this function with regard to literature:

> For we are apt to forget, reading, as we tend to do, only the masterpieces of a bygone age how great a power the body of literature possesses to impose itself: how it will not suffer itself to be read passively, but takes us and reads us; flouts our preconceptions; questions principles which we had got into the habit of taking for granted, and, in fact, splits us into two parts as we read, making us, even as we enjoy, yield our ground or stick to our guns. (1925/1953, 49)

When one is moved by the existence and autonomy of imaginal others and their worlds, one often experiences a luminous or religious quality to these dialogues; one comes upon prayer. The symbolic possibilities of imaginal dialogues are most highly developed in poetry, novels and plays, but are present in our fantasy as well.

A Phenomenon is not Pathological in and of Itself but with Respect to a Given Telos *and Context*

But of course not all imaginal dialogues would be means to these dramatic, symbolic, or spiritual ends. Clinicians know that some such dialogues can have an obsessive and repetitive quality that monopolizes thought without taking it further. Other such dialogues are confused with perception. Some are hallucinatory in character. Others are examples of extreme egocentricity, where all the characters are known shallowly or only from the point of view of the ego. Our task will be to specify the kinds of imaginal dialogues that would be means to the *teloi* specified, and in so doing to take up the issue of pathological dialogues—those that would not further these ends. Once again the *teloi* and the context—just as they pick out some changes in childhood to be developmental and not others—also pick out what is to be considered pathological and what is not. A particular kind of imaginal dialogue is not pathological in and of itself, but only with respect to the given *telos* and context.

The Universalizing of a Given Telos

Theorists and their readers tend to universalize the *telos* under discussion. We have seen this in Piaget's case where logic dominates the discussion of rather diverse phenomena, and in psychoanalysis where adaptation to "reality" holds full sway. In the former case the child is seen as a budding scientist, coming to fully recognize the necessity of "conforming to the intellectual structures of logic, Euclidean geometry, and the other basic Kantian forms" (Toulmin, 1981, 256). If we were to substitute for Piaget's goal for thought, the *telos* of the child becoming a budding dramatist, the "facts" we would read would differ from Piaget, Vygotsky, and Mead's. For instance, from a dramatic perspective how would we re-see their developmental theories? Vygotsky's elliptical internal monologues might be seen not as monologues, but as dialogues having the formal features of speech with an intimate other. Mead's "generalized other" might be seen not as an absence of a specific imaginal other to whom thoughts are directed, but as denoting that the thought/speech, while being directed to a specific imaginal other, is formed in a way that is understandable to a large audience. Or finally, Piaget's thesis that the dialogues in play develop into abstract thought might be understood not as evidence of the absence of imaginal dialogues in adult life, but as a consequence of the growing child's identification with the role of being a scientist. Early imaginal dialogues would then be seen not only as stepping stones to abstract thought or social discourse, but as expressive of the dramatic quality of mind (a thesis with many roots in philosophy, religion, aesthetics, and the early history of psychiatry).[17] This point of view presupposes a re-valuation of the role of imagination in mental life.

Conclusion

Instead of proposing a single line of development for imaginal dialogues, we are suggesting that there are several; which one is observed will depend on the chosen *telos*. We are not satisfied with the conclusion that all such dialogues become communicative speech or abstract thought. This leads to the implicit evaluation of imaginal dialogues as inferior processes which are gradually overcome in favor of more adequate communication or more logical and abstract thought. Nor shall we rest with a single line of development from the specific characters of childhood play to the generalized other, denuded of particular character or costume, homogenized and neatened for the purposes of adult thought. We shall focus on the development of imaginal dialogues, not their disappearance or their inadequacy. Our attention will therefore not be directed to the dissolution of imaginal others as they are assimilated into a broader "ego" or "self" through acts of interpretation. Rather, we will be concerned with the development of the imaginal other from an extension of the ego, a passive recipient of the imaginer's intention, to an autonomous and animate agency in its own right. We will be less concerned with the development of a "generalized" nature of a sole imaginal other, and more concerned with the deepening of characterization of many imaginal others. We will not dwell on how the imaginal other is really ourself, but pursue further how the imaginal other is gradually

---

[17] We are contrasting a scientifically oriented, logical, abstract thought to a poetic and dramatic one, the former tending toward monologues, the latter toward dialogue. This might also be described not as a contrast between males and females, but between masculine and feminine forms of thought. In the feminine form, others are always taken into account. The agent does not imagine him or herself as at the center (Hermann, 1981, 88). Thought in this instance is either dialogical or at the boarder of dialogue—occurring as it does in the interstices of the personal. This organization of self in relation to others can be contrasted with thought that has a single, dominant voice, around which all else centers at any given moment. This is akin to Gilligan's (1982) contrast between a masculine form of morality where abstract principles are applied across situations, and a feminine form where the agent becomes immersed imaginatively in the particular points of view within a given situation in order to come to a determination (again more implicitly dialogical).

released from our egocentrism to an autonomy from which he or she creates us as much as we create him or her. We will acknowledge the experience of our identity shifting back and forth between various personae. However this acknowledgment will not lead us only to the familiar claim that all imaginal others should be not only understood as but also experienced as aspects of self. Rather we shall look at how the self develops through both the experience of being in dialogue with imaginal others who are felt as autonomous, and the experience of even the "I" as being in flux between various characterizations.

From this perspective, personifying is seen as a human propensity not limited to children, members of "primitive" cultures, or cases of psychopathology. It is fundamental not only to mythology, poetry, drama, literature, and religion, but to thought itself. Imaginal dialogues are one of a number of possible transactions with those imaginal "personified" others who arise either spontaneously—as in early play, conversations in thought or dreams—or through a form of practice such as Jung's active imagination, or the writing of fiction or poetry.

PART III

*Re-Conceiving a Developmental Theory
of Imaginal Dialogues*

CHAPTER SEVEN

"The Characters Speak Because They Want to Speak:"
The Autonomy of the Imaginal Other

> One cannot "make" characters, only marionettes.
> —Elizabeth Bowen, 1975

> ...the characters speak because they want
> To speak, the fat, the roseate characters,
> Free, for a moment, from malice and sudden cry,
> Complete in a completed scene, speaking
> Their parts as in a youthful happiness.
> —Wallace Stevens, from "Credences of Summer"

In a secular world, whose boundaries and dimensions are drawn by those who accept the structures of science as God-given rules, the concept of projection has been used to locate in a shadowy interior of "mind" all those experiences which can find no place in the so-called "objective" order of things. And so, inevitably, for those who would make current science sacred, the imaginal other is believed to be an aspect of self or of the self's experience which is projected outward and given a personified form. This may be so.

But just when we begin to treat all characters of the imagination as mere projections of self, a central paradox emerges. Although the other may bear some resemblance to myself or my experience, this is not always the case. I often do not plan his appearance. In the midst of my thinking, my activities, my speaking, I find he has appeared and spoken to me. In some cases, I cannot predict what he will say or know when he will end. It is true that it is my awareness which occasions my noting of him but, apart from that, the imaginal other may have as much autonomy as the so-called real others I meet in consensual space. If one insists that, in theory, I created him, it can with equal force be maintained that, in experience, it seems as though he created me. "The songs made me, not I them," said Goethe. Even if one accepts that I have created him, one must also acknowledge that this creation, like the procreation of a child, leads to my offspring's existing independently of my conscious intention.

I say "often" and not "always" because one can consciously conjure up a character and deny her autonomy, carefully lending her only one's own words and desired qualities. However when setting about this attempt to cabin, crib, and confine, one can often catch oneself suppressing actions, phrases, and characteristics that threaten to assert themselves outside one's conscious intention. Elizabeth Bowen, speaking of the creation of a novel, said, "The term 'creation of character' (or characters) is misleading. Characters preexist, they are found" (1975, 172). A similar ambiguity concerning "invention" and "discovery" is found among mathematicians and philosophers of mathematics. Do mathematicians invent their remarkable structures or do they discover them? The paradox is compounded when one realizes that to invent originally meant "to find out," "to discover." The interpenetrating of fact and fiction suggested by their common linguistic root is surely at the heart of the philosophical ambiguity.

Among those who have most profoundly challenged the scientistic and reductionistic attempt to denature and de-realize those objects of experience that do not fit neatly into the scientific construction of reality is the philosopher Ernst Cassirer. In his critical examination of those reductionistic conceptions of the structure and function of the mythic world, Cassirer argues against all attempts to "twist the world of objective change back into the subjective world and interpret it according to the categories of the subjective world."

> For man does not simply transfer his own finished personality to the god or simply lend him his own feeling and consciousness of himself: it is rather through the figure of his gods that man first finds this self-consciousness. (Cassirer, 1955, 155, 211)

THE AUTONOMY OF THE IMAGINAL OTHER 95

The articulation of the imaginal other is at the same time an articulation of the being and activity of the self. These articulations are not only aimed at establishing a rudimentary sense of self but are an ongoing and changing way of participating in the complex meanings and correlative definitions of self and world.

Cassirer emphasizes how in mythical consciousness, even if a tutelary spirit is closely associated with a person—perhaps even believed to inhabit his body or govern his being—this spirit is conceived of not

> ...as the man's I, as the "subject" of his inner life, but as something objective, which dwells in man, which is spatially connected with him and hence can also be spatially separated from him... And even where the closest possible relation exists between the tutelary spirit and the man in whom it dwells...it nevertheless appears as something existing for itself, something separate and strange. (1955, 168)

For example, the Bataks of Sumatra hold the belief that it is a spirit which determines the character and fortune of a person. The spirit is like a man within a man, but it "does not coincide with his personality and is often in conflict with his I; it is a special being within the man, having its own will and its own desires, which it is able to gratify against the man's will and to the man's discomfiture" (Warneck, 1909, 8).

Experiences of this sort are not confined to times past and cultures far away. We need only turn to novelists' experiences with their characters.[18] According to the novelist, painter, and aesthetician Joyce Cary, when Proust was writing *Remembrance of Things Past*, a woman, Mme. Schiff, wrote Proust to complain that his character Swann had become ridiculous. Proust, Cary says, responded that he (Proust) "had no wish to make Swann ridiculous, far from it. But when he had come to this part of the work, he had found it unavoidable." In his

---

[18] Although painters often work from form and color as much as from imagined beings, these too are often experienced as presences which suggest themselves to the artist from outside. For instance, Miro said that "forms take reality for me as I work. In other words, rather than setting out to paint something, I begin painting and as I paint the picture begins to assert itself, or suggest something under my brush." For Nolde, forms were vehicles for color, "Color in their own lives," "weeping and laughing, dream and bliss, hot and sacred, like love songs and the erotic like songs and glorious chorale! Colors in vibration, pealing like silver bells and clanging like bronze bells, proclaiming happiness, passion, and love, soul, blood and death" (quoted in *The Smithsonian*, January, 1981).

jealousy, Swann acted in the "ridiculous way he did in spite of Proust's intention as author." Cary explains,

> It is a form of intuition; it is the immediate recognition of a real truth, a penetration into the realities of character. And it has broken through Proust's first conception of Swann, and immediately deepened his awareness of Swann's possibilities. Swann, as a character created by Proust, here assumes an individual personality to be intuited by his own author. (1958, 87-88)

Cary presents another example of a character so autonomous that the intensity of his words and beliefs radically alters the author's intentions for him: Ivan in *The Brothers Karamazov*. Dostoevsky's famous "Pro and Contra" chapter, rather than asserting the inadequacies of atheism compared with orthodoxy, as Dostoevsky had originally intended, did just the reverse.

> [When Dostoevsky] asked himself how would Ivan see reality, how would he argue about it, he realised with the force of intuition a truth that had been before only the statement of a hypothetical case, and then expressed it with the utmost power. So that his scheme for that chapter, his concept *a priori* of what that chapter would mean, was completely ruined. (Cary, 1958, 85)

Ivan's arguments arise independently of Dostoevsky's desire. Indeed, as Cary points out, Dostoevsky was "terrified:"

> He feared the Government censors. He wrote to all his religious and orthodox friends to tell them that in the very next installment he would bring in his priest, the saintly Father Zossima, to answer Ivan. He spent weeks on those fifty pages which were to give the refutation. And, after all his work, he failed most dismally. (41)

This experience of autonomy appears to be true as well for characters based on real life people. Eugene O'Neill (1981) claimed he had never written about a character who was not an actual person. "But, " he was quick to add, "even these things have a way of developing!"

Marina Tsvetaeva, an early twentieth-century Russian poet, described how she was moved to write by the imaginal being "which wanted to exist through" her. The hand of an artist, she said, belongs not to oneself but to that being. In a letter to Pasternak, Tsvetaeva said, "We dream and write not when we please but when it pleases" (quoted in Muchnic, 1980, 7). She would often experience herself writing against her own will, motivated instead by the beings that chose her to give them life.[19] The poet Joseph Brodsky compared Tsvetaeva's poetry to folklore, saying that she spoke not in a "heroine's monologue" but in a "shepherd's song," in "speech intended for one's self, for one's own being," when "the speaker is also his own hearer" and "the ear listens to the mouth" (quoted in Muchnic, 1980).

Certainly not all authors experience their characters forcing them to write against their will (what psychiatry calls a delusion of influence). Not even Tsvetaeva experienced that all the time. Nor do we experience imaginal others as always having this high degree of autonomy. What I am pointing to is a continuum ranging from the imaginal other's having no thoughts, feelings, or actions which the conscious self does not lend it to the imaginal other's acting, feeling and speaking in ways that surprise the self. Take for example the following experience of the novelist Francine du Plessis Gray (quoted in Christy, 1981).

> I know the characters personally. They are sleeping in my bed with me. They wake me. They demand and insist on knowing what I am going to do with them next. I can let loose in my writing, make an alternate world that stands next to the real one. I can create the characters I would have liked to have been.

This example is intermediate in the sense that the characters are capable of initiating actions—they wake one, demand and insist— and yet the author is in charge of what happens to them next, who they are to become.

On either side of this example we can find Sartre and Mauriac engaged in a debate about the role of the author in modern literature. The debate concerns whether the author takes an omniscient role with respect to the characters, knowing all their actions, thoughts and feelings and delivering these to the reader. Sartre argues that Mauriac himself sat in the center of his heroine's consciousness, helping her "lie to herself and, at the same time, judging and condemning her" (quoted in Harvey, 1965, 163). Mauriac, says Sartre,

---

[19] Guy de Maupassant saw his double sitting at the other side of his writing desk and would hear his double dictating what he should write (Rogers, 1970).

> wrote that the novelist is to his own creatures what God is to His. And that explains all the oddities of his technique. He takes God's standpoint on his characters. God sees the inside and outside, the depths of body and soul, the whole universe at once. In like manner, M. Mauriac is omniscient about everything relating to his little world. What he says about his characters is Gospel... The time has come to say that the novelist is not God. (quoted in Harvey, 1965, 163)

Sartre asks Mauriac, "Do you want your characters to live?... See to it that they are free" (162).

He might also have asked this of George Sand, whose method of putting her words into the mouths of her characters contradicts her stated intention that they not be like dolls.

> He obeys my every whim, my mood, my will...all his movements are the consequences of my own thoughts and my own words which I have put into his mouth...he is "me," in short, a human being and not just a doll. (quoted in Rambert, 1949, 1)

Had she known Jean Paul Richter or Sartre, they probably would have fought. It was Richter who said,

> A poet who must reflect whether he shall make a character say yes or no—to the devil with him; he is only a stupid corpse. (quoted in Darwin, 1871)

Sartre was intent on wanting "to drive providence from our works as we have driven it from our world." In place of the god-like author, Sartre wished to

> find an orchestration of consciousnesses which may permit us to render the multidimensionality of the event. Moreover, in giving up the fiction of the omniscient narrator, we have assumed the obligation of suppressing the intermediaries between the reader and the subjectivities. It is a matter of having him enter into their minds as into a windmill. (quoted in Harvey 1965, 162, 164)

Enid Blyton describes how, in the process of writing, her characters let her know what is going on, rather than the other way around.

> I shut my eyes for a few moments, with my portable typewriter on my knee—I make my mind blank and wait—

THE AUTONOMY OF THE IMAGINAL OTHER

> and then, as clearly as I would see real children, my characters stand before me in my mind's eye. I see them in detail—hair, eyes, feet, clothes, expression—and I always know their Christian names, but never their surnames... I don't know what anyone is going to say or do. I don't know what is going to happen. I am in the happy position of being able to write a story and read it for the first time, at one and the same moment... Sometimes a character makes a joke, a really funny one, that makes me laugh as I type it on my paper—and I think, "Well, I couldn't have thought of that myself in a hundred years!" And then I think, "Well, who did think of it, then?"
> (quoted in Stoney, 1974)

We see development from one end toward the other of this continuum of dependence-autonomy in children's early relations to their dolls. At first the imaginal other is an egocentric extension of one's habitual stance. The other is not allowed an autonomy, often not even an attributed or projected interiority. The child puts the doll to bed and pretends to read it a story. The doll is not lent or allowed animation of its own but is rather the prop of the imaginer's intention to be a caretaker. And this phenomenon is not restricted to children. The puppet-like status of the imaginal other may easily be found in imaginal transactions in adulthood as well. The imaginer may speak to an imaginal child but allow it no response. The feelings of the child may be assumed by the imaginer, but never is the child asked, nor are her spontaneous expressions noted (if even allowed for at all). The absence of autonomy can result in repetitive fantasies; only one point of view is being played out.

How different this is from experiences in which one does not know how the characters and their scenarios will unfold, in which the novel and the ego-alien appear and develop. Henry James, in his preface to *The Ambassadors*, described how the book arose from an anecdote told him at a garden party in Paris. The anecdote concerned an older man telling a younger one about his philosophy of life. This was to become the central scene of a book. "But what else?" James asked himself.

> Where has he come from this older man and why has he come, what is he doing... To answer these questions plausibly, to answer them as under cross-examination in the witness box by counsel for the prosecution, in other words

> to satisfactorily account for the character Strether and for his "peculiar tone" was to possess myself of the entire fabric. (1934, 313)

Now listen to James describing himself in relation to the development of this novel.

> These things continued to fall together, as by the neat action of their own weight and form even while their commentator James himself scratched his head about them; he easily sees now that they were always well in advance of him. As the case completed itself he had in fact, from a good way behind, to catch up with them; breathless and a little flurried, as he best could. (1934, 315)

Similarly, Flannery O'Connor[20] in her essay, "Writing Short Stories," speaks of how she often did not know where she was going when she sat down to write a short story. She cites the experience of writing "Good Country People" as an example of how her writing was like discovery.

> When I started writing that story, I didn't know there was going to be a Ph.D. with a wooden leg in it. I merely found myself one morning writing a description of two women I knew something about, and before I realized it, I had equipped one of them with a daughter with a wooden leg. As the story progressed, I brought in the Bible salesman, but I had no idea what I was going to do with him. I didn't know he was going to steal that wooden leg until ten or twelve lines before he did it, but when I found out that this was what was going to happen, I realized that it was inevitable. (1961, 100)[21]

O'Connor says that nothing can be predicted about these mysterious moments in a story, for "they represent the working of grace for the characters" (116).

For Alice Walker the writing of the novel *The Color Purple* entailed a year of speaking with Celie and Shug and the other characters. She

---

[20] For other such examples, see Cary (1958, 127-134) and Carver (1981, 18).

[21] O'Connor continues: "As soon as the writer 'learns to write,' as soon as he knows what he is going to find, and discovers a way to say what he knew all along, or worse still, a way to say nothing, he is finished. If a writer is any good, what he makes will have its source in a realm much larger than that which his conscious mind can encompass and will always be a greater surprise to him than it can ever be to his reader" (1961, 83).

experienced them as "trying to contact" her, "to speak through her" (1983, 357). These presences did not ignore Walker's day to day life. Indeed, they pressured her to move from the city to the country, expressed opinions about her work-life, and enjoyed a relation to her daughter. They offered other perspectives on situations than the ones Walker identified with.

> Just as summer was ending, one or more of my characters—Celie, Shug, Albert, Sofia, or Harpo—would come for a visit. We would sit wherever I was, and talk. They were very obliging, engaging, and jolly. They were, of course, at the end of their story but were telling it to me from the beginning. Things that made me sad, often made them laugh. Oh, we got through that; don't pull such a long face, they'd say. Or, you think Reagan's bad, you ought've seen some of the rednecks us come up under. The days passed in a blaze of happiness. (359)

Within academic and clinical psychology, the autonomy of such characters has been relegated primarily to discussions of hallucinations, hysterical dissociations, split personalities. The non-pathological experience of the autonomy of imaginal others—as in the examples above—is neither dealt with in itself or allowed to influence clinical theory. There are some notable exceptions to this generalization, however (see Watkins, 1984). Let us approach Jung as one of these. Jung began his psychiatric career working in the asylum, surrounding himself with the voices and visions of patients' psychoses. Rather than relegating the experience of imaginal figures to the limbo of pathology, he actively sought his own voices. This led him to his researches in the history of mythology, religion and alchemy. In these domains, Jung found support for his theory that imaginal figures are not necessarily evidence of pathology, but are indicative of the process of personification that occurs spontaneously in the "unconscious."

Jung argues that it is not we who personify these figures but they who "have a personal nature from the beginning" (1968a, § 62). He tries to account for their autonomy with his notion of archetypes. The figures are not considered mere projections but issue from nonpersonal archetypes, from formative dispositions. The individual characters one experiences are both expressions of one's ego and life and also variations on forms which exist independently of the person. In this way Jung accounts for the experience of the figures' autonomy and his observation of parallels in imagery across time and place.

When Jung engaged the imaginal figures that appeared to him in dialogue—such as Philemon—he directly experienced their autonomy.

> Philemon and other figures of my fantasies brought home to me the crucial insight that there are things in the psyche which I do not produce, but which produce themselves and have their own life. Philemon represented a force which was not myself. In my fantasies I held conversations with him, and he said things which I had not consciously thought. For I observed clearly that it was he who spoke, not I. He said I treated thoughts as if I generated them myself, but in his view thoughts were like animals in the forest, or people in a room, or birds in the air, and added, "If you should see people in a room, you would not think that you made these people, or that you were responsible for them." It was he who taught me psychic objectivity, the reality of the psyche. Through him the distinction was clarified between myself and the object of my thought. He confronted me in an objective manner, and I understood that there is something in me which can say things that I do not know and do not intend, things which may even be directed against me.
>
> Psychologically, Philemon represented superior insight. He was a mysterious figure to me. At times he seemed to me quite real, as if he were a living personality. I went walking up and down the garden with him, and to me he was what the Indians call a guru. (Jung, 1961, § 183)

Whether we accept the theory of archetypes and Jung's idea that "there are things in the psyche" that one does not produce, these are attempts to have theory conform to experience, rather than the other way around (as often, but not always, happens in psychoanalytic theory). This conformity of theory with experience involves Jung, on the one hand, in creating explanatory principles which have yet to be widely accepted. On the other hand, it leads to a set of therapeutic procedures which encourage one to pursue experiences with imaginal figures in the manner that they present themselves—to relate to them as autonomous.

Jung calls the process of engaging figures and images, coming to form a conscious relation to them, "active imagination." He understands this process as an ancient one with many parallels in history.

THE AUTONOMY OF THE IMAGINAL OTHER 103

> In antiquity when a man had to direct a prayer to the statue of the god, he stepped upon a stone that was erected at its side to enable people to shout their prayer into the ear, so that the god would hear them, and then he stared at the image until the god nodded his head or opened or shut his eyes or answered in some way. You see this was an abbreviated method of active imagination, concentrating upon the image until it moved; and in that moment the god gave a hint, his assent or his denial or any other indication, and that is the numinosum. (Jung, 1937, 2)

Henry Miller describes just this sort of experience, albeit secularized:

> Occasionally this same sort of bitchery would start up with statues, particularly chipped and dismantled ones. I might be loitering in some backyard gazing absentmindedly at a marble head with one ear missing and presto! it would be talking to me...talking in the language of a proconsul. Some crazy urge would seize me to caress the battered features, whereupon, as if the touch of my hand had restored it to life, it would smile at me. Then an even stranger thing might happen. An hour later, say, passing the plate glass window of an empty shop, who would greet me from the murky depths but the same proconsul! Terror stricken, I would press my nose against the shop-window and stare. There he was—an ear missing, the nose bitten off. And his lips moving! "A retinal hemorrhage," I would murmur, and move on. "God help me if he visits me in my sleep!" (1939, 10)

In a letter to a Mr. O, Jung described the process of active imagination this way:

> The point is that you start with any image, for instance, with just that yellow mass in your dream. Contemplate it and carefully observe how the picture begins to unfold or to change. Don't try to make it into something, just do nothing but observe what its spontaneous changes are. Any mental picture you contemplate in this way will sooner or later change through a spontaneous association that causes a slight alteration of the picture. You must carefully avoid impatient jumping from one subject to another. Hold fast to the one image you have chosen and wait until it changes by itself, and if it is a speaking figure

at all then say what you have to say to that figure and listen to what he or she has to say. (1973, 459-460)

If we approach the imaginal other as a projection resulting from a defensive refusal to recognize certain qualities, feelings or wishes in oneself—i.e., if we approach it from the point of view of our usual psychoanalytic causal explanations—then the therapeutic move involves a process of reclamation, whereby the ego attempts to recognize, claim, and assimilate the psychic fragments which have appeared in personified form. There is a widening of the ego as a multiplicity of figures are absorbed and de-personified. From this point of view the persistent autonomy of imaginal others is a negative or pathological phenomenon. Recall Schafer's admonition:

> Too often, introjects are written about (and discussed in the clinic) as if they were actual persons carrying on lives of their own, with energies of their own, and with independent intentions directed toward the subject.
>
> ...[T]hey should be treated merely as thoughts, ideas, or information... For theory to portray representations in any other way is to verge on an implicit demonology and not to build an internally consistent and parsimonious psychology. (1968, 83, 138-139)

Schafer certainly advocates an omniscient ego role and a de-personification of psychic life, and his moves in therapy through action language are meant to encourage this (see Schafer, 1976, 155-178).

While some imaginal figures are clearly personifications of rejected possibilities for the self, can we account for all of them in this way? Moreover, even if the self gains distance by dislocation and personification of psychic possibilities, would not an intense reciprocal dialogue with the resulting imaginal figures ultimately mitigate their supposed defensive function by requiring the self to come to terms with them as partners in dialogue?

If we approach the experience of imaginal dialogues by valuing the dramatic quality of mind which gives rise to imaginal worlds, then the interpretive and explanatory moves which result from projection theory and which aim at de-personifying and de-potentiating these figures become problematic. When the dramatic quality of mind is valued, a different set of moves aimed at developing this quality must be proposed. Such moves need not invite a demonology.

If we begin, as Jung did, with a respect for the imaginal other that sees the presence of a figure as a non-pathological occurrence (i.e., that views personifying as a spontaneous process not always serving a defensive function), then the activities of the imagining ego need not be de-personification, de-potentiation, reclamation, assimilation—but instead the building of relationships in dialogue. The self does not attempt to abolish the autonomous presence of the other. Development does not coincide with a move from presence to absence, from projection to assimilation, integrating the voices and figures. Rather development occurs in the dialogue between self and other, in the process of mutual articulation.

And it is dialogue that we find wherever autonomy is granted. Whether we note how Egyptians spoke to their *Ba*, Homeric men to their *thumos*,[22] Henry Miller to his characters, or Jung to Philemon, dialogue is the consistent activity. "Dialogue is the ideal means of showing what is between the characters. It crystallizes relationship," says Elizabeth Bowen (1975, 180).

We have focused on the experienced autonomy[23] of the characters: the experiences of their initiating interactions, of their seeming to have lives apart from the ego, of their affecting the ego, creating the ego, as much as the ego them. In using the term "autonomy" I make no claim that such characters exist in objectified nature, in and of themselves, independently of their being experienced. Nor do I mean that their apprehended qualities are independent of their relationship with a particular ego.

I am, however, stressing that whereas psychological theory which values "abstract" thought would most often see changes from autonomy to dependence, de-personification, and assimilation as positive developments, theory which values "dramatic" thought would encourage a development toward autonomy of characters. Similarly, we find that theorists who reduce the development of thought to the development of abstract thought propose that the early multiplicity

---

[22] "A man's *thumos* tells him that he must now eat or drink or slay an enemy, it advises him on the course of his action, it puts words into his mouth... He can converse with it, or with his 'heart' or his 'belly,' almost as man to man. Sometimes he scolds these detached entities, ususally he takes their advice, but he may also reject it" (Dodds, 1951, 16).

[23] See Casey (1976b, 175-234) for a discussion on how imagining itself can be seen as an autonomous act.

of specific characters in childhood play become, by adulthood, homogenized into a single voice, the "generalized other" as described by George Herbert Mead. The idea that characters become not only more autonomous but also more highly specified and discrete in their identities goes against the grain of much of developmental theory. But is it not precisely the particularity of characters that helps differentiate the multiplicity of perspectives which is so critical to the development of thought as well as literature and myth?

CHAPTER EIGHT

The Dialogues Between Multiple Characters: The Monologues of Multiple Personality

*I cannot understand the mystery but
I am always conscious of myself as two.
Do I contradict myself?
Very well then I contradict myself,
I am large, I contain multitudes.* —Walt Whitman

*There never was...a good biography of a good novelist.
There couldn't be. He's too many people if he's any good.*
—F. Scott Fitzgerald (quoted in Rogers, 1970)

Whereas psychoanalytic and developmental theories advocate a developmental unification of the various imaginal personae over time, a perspective which valued dramatic thought would struggle to maintain multiplicity. Contrary to fearful expectation, this multiplicity of characters in an individual's experience would not resemble a pathological state of "multiple personality." In the latter there is no imaginal dialogue, only sequential monologue. The person identifies with or is taken over by various characters in a sequential fashion. The ego is most often unaware of the other voices. It is paradoxical that the illness of multiple personality is problematic precisely because of its singleness of voice at any one moment, not because of its multiplicity. Improvement starts when dialogue and reflection between the selves begins to happen, when there is multiplicity in a single moment of time, rather than multiplicity over time (see Schreiber, 1973).

The multiplicity we are advocating from a dramatic point of view is one where the characters are in dialogue. Why? What virtue do we see in multiplicity? This is like asking what were the virtues of polytheism, or of the experience of multiple souls prevalent in many earlier cultures. The questions are analogous because in all three cases an individual relates to a multiplicity of figures, and experiences him or herself and the world through this multiplicity of selves, gods, or souls. The rejection of polytheism can be likened, as it has been by Hillman (1971), to the rejection of a polycentric psyche.

In the history of religions and in ethnology there have been moves to see monotheism as a developmental advance over polytheism. Scholars such as Paul Radin (1954) have argued that such supposed developmental facts need to be called into question. In his monograph on "Monotheism among primitive people" (1954; quoted in Hillman, 1971, 794) Radin rejects an evolutionary view and argues that "as most ethnologists and unbiased students would now admit, the possibility of interpreting monotheism as part of a general intellectual and ethical progress must be abandoned." Cassirer also argues that a multiplicity of souls and gods is not only found in elementary forms of myth, but even in more "advanced configurations...the motif of the soul's division far overbalances that of its unity" (1955, 163).

In discussing the function and virtue of this multiplicity in other, earlier cultures, Cassirer illuminates the virtues of a multiplicity of imaginal figures in our own experience:

> In the multiplicity of his gods man not only merely beholds the outward diversity of natural objects and forces but also perceives himself in the concrete diversity and distinction of his functions. The countless gods he makes for himself guide him not only through the sphere of objective reality and change but above all through the sphere of his own will and accomplishment, which they illumine from within. He becomes aware of the trend peculiar to each concrete activity only by viewing it objectively in the image of the special god belonging to it. Action is differentiated into distinct independent functions not through abstract discursive concept formation but by the contrary process, wherein each of these functions is apprehended as an intuitive whole and embodied in an independent mythical figure. (1955, 203-204)

In other words the multiplicity of souls could be successive in time or simultaneous, a person might receive a new soul at different life transitions or have more than one soul throughout life. Cassirer goes on to say:

> for mythical thinking the same splitting process can be successive as well as coexistent: just as very different "souls" can live peacefully side by side in one and the same man, so the empirical sequence of the events of life can be distributed among wholly different "subjects," each of which is not only *thought* in the form of a separate being, but also *felt* and *intuited* as a living demonic power which takes possession of the man. (1955, 165)

Here multiplicity is viewed not as a fragmentation or splitting of a unity—as in psychoanalysis—but as a process of differentiation. Each imaginal figure provides a different perspective through which events and the self itself can be viewed. We readily acknowledge the virtue of this multiplicity in literature and drama, but distance ourselves from it when it is suggested as a personal experience. We would not judge a play or novel with one character as necessarily better or worse than another with several characters. So why should we impose this kind of ideal on the richness of our own thought?[24]

In the tradition of psychology, the notion of multiplicity reared its head in discussions of spiritism and hysteria in the second half of the nineteenth century. At that time Flournoy, Janet, Myers, Jung, and others noted how the personhood of the hysteric or medium would be as though given over to another whose ways of speaking, moving, thinking and valuing might be wholly inconsistent with the person with whom the observer had been familiar. These observations led to two distinct notions about multiplicity which have since been consistently confused: 1) multiplicity as symptomatic of disease; and 2) multiplicity as an inherent result of the mythopoetic nature of mind (see Watkins, 1974). From the latter point of view, it was argued that it was not multiplicity of imaginal others that was pathognomic, but rather the co-presence of other factors such as the de-differentiation of the perceptual and the imaginal, the disowning of relation to the

---

[24] In therpy we can sometimes follow the course of how one character becomes two. Often this proliferation does not result from a lack of integration, but issues from a high degree of differentiation, of characterization. For example, see the case presented in Chapter Twelve.

imaginal others, over-identification with one figure, or a lack of awareness of figures. Personifying was a universal tendency of mind that did not in itself bode illness. From this point of view multiplicity of imaginal figures was viewed positively, as yielding imaginal backgrounds that specifically symbolized the multiplicity of life experiences and activities. Just as dreams bring before us multiple characters, so it was felt that such figures are close at hand when we feel or think, or even perceive; when we love, fight, or desire.

The acceptance of multiplicity as a fact of psychic life has far exceeded the valuing of multiplicity. Within orthodox psychoanalysis, multiplicity is synonymous with "fragmentation." In more popular forms of psychotherapy (psychodrama, gestalt therapy, psychosynthesis, transactional analysis, guided imagery) as well as in some forms of behavior modification (see Meichenbaum and Goodman, 1979), multiplicity is accepted and this acknowledgment opens the door to a variety of treatment techniques. Yet the prescribed developmental course is often from the many to the one, from imaginal to solely historical reality.

Our intellectual tradition sees an ego-centered psyche just as it sees monotheism; not only as a later achievement but a better one than a polycentered psyche and polytheism. As Jung said,

> If tendencies towards dissociation were not inherent in the human psyche, fragmentary psychic systems would never have been split off; in other words, neither spirits nor gods would have ever come into existence. That is also the reason why our time has become so utterly godless and profane: we lack all knowledge of the unconscious psyche and pursue the cult of consciousness to the exclusion of all else. Our true religion is a monotheism of consciousness, a possession by it, coupled with a fanatical denial of the existence of fragmentary autonomous systems. (1969a, § 51)

But even Jung, whose psychology was most firmly based on a polycentric notion of psyche, emphasized that the culmination of development was the emergence of the Self, an admittedly monotheistic-like idea (Hillman, 1971). Jung described psyche as a multiplicity of partial consciousnesses (see Jung, 1969, 338*ff*). Drawing on the imagery of the alchemists, he likened psyche to a star-strewn night sky with multiple planets and constellations (Paracelsus) or of fish eyes glimmering in a dark sea like gold (Morienus Romanus). In his system these stars or planets were called complexes, and each complex acted autonomously from the ego and presented itself in the imaginal persons of dreams and fantasies. A prime concern of Jung's opus was to sort out the multiplicity of imaginal figures which occur not only in modern dreams and waking dreams, but also in mythology, religion and literature. For him the parallels between figures arising from these different sources were evidence for the existence of archetypes. As we have seen, object relations theorists have also sorted such figures into different categories arising from radically different conceptions about the etiology and status of imaginal figures: good and bad objects (Klein); exciting, rejecting, and ideal objects; libidinal, antilibidinal and central egos (Fairbaim); sadomasochistic oral and passive aggressive egos (Guntrip).

In Hillman's work[25] the "monotheistic" treatment of these dramatic personae (i.e., the kind of treatment that sponsors unity over multiplicity) is brought fully into question. He argues that the usual emphasis on integrating the multiplicity of figures into a wholeness ought to be balanced by a careful differentiation of this wholeness into specific figures. This move to multiplicity is not the same as encouraging dissociation and confusion. Like monotheistic conceptions, it too has its order. This lies in the differentiation of the figures and the manner of relations formed with them.

Kaplan and Crockett (1968) warn that to have unity in diversity one needs a hierarchization which while preserving the differences, modulates and coordinates them as well. One may fail to achieve unity in diversity through merely juxtaposing or sequentializing the diversity (separation without integration) or through collapsing the plurality (syncretism). With respect to imaginal figures the focus would be on the relations between the voices. As in a play one figure does not simply speak after another or while another is speaking, but acts and speaks in relation to the others and to the emerging patterns of significance that make the various scenes cohere.

Biologist Lewis Thomas makes a similar observation in a humorous piece on the multiplicity of imaginal figures:

---

[25] For Hillman's treatment of polytheism and monotheism with respect to psyche, see the following: 1971, 1972 (265), 1975b (26, 127, 167, 193, 226). Also see Kaplan and Crockett's (1968) treatment of the theme of unity and diversity and Miller (1974).

> Odd to say, it is not just a jumble of talk; they tend to space what they're saying so that words and phrases from one will fit into short spaces left in silence by the others. At good times it has the feel of an intensely complicated conversation, but at others the sounds are more like something overheard in a crowded station. At worse times the silences get out of synchrony, interrupting each other; it is as though all the papers had suddenly blown off the table. (1974, 43-44)

Thomas questions whether the number of different selves is in itself pathological. He hopes not and argues the following:

> It is the simultaneity of their appearance that is the real problem, and I think psychiatry would do better by simply persuading them to queue up and wait their turn, as happens in the normal rest of us...

> Actually, it would embarrass me to be told that more than a single self is a kind of disease. I've had, in my time, more than I could possibly count or keep track of. The great difference, which keeps me feeling normal, is that mine (ours) have turned up one after the other... The only thing close to what you might call illness, in my experience, was in the gaps in the queue when one had finished and left the place before the next one was ready to start, and there was nobody around at all. (42)

CHAPTER NINE

Character Development:
The Articulation of the Imaginal Other

A character is interesting as it comes out and by the process and duration of that emergence; just as a procession is effective by the way it unfolds, turning into a mere mob if it all passes at once.
—Henry James

Tolstoy criticized Gorky: "Most of what you say comes out of yourself, and therefore you have no characters, and all your people have the same face." —Tolstoy (quoted in Gorky, 1946, 21)

Tolstoy shares with Gorky his knowledge that when one does not allow characters their autonomy, one merely projects from oneself, lending them one's own face. When one allows characters to speak, to be known apart from the self, then a depth and specificity of characterization can develop.

Similarly, in *The Common Reader* (1925) Virginia Woolf discusses the difference between Elizabethan drama and the modern novel. In the former, she claims, there were no real characters. For instance, in Ford's *'Tis Pity She's A Whore*, we gropingly come to know that the character Annabella

> …is a spirited girl, with her defiance of her husband when he abuses her, her snatches of Italian song, her ready wit, her simple glad love-making. But of character as we understand the word there is no trace. We do not know how she reaches her conclusions, only that she has reached

> them. Nobody describes her. She is always at the height of her passion, never at its approach. Compare her with Anna Karenina. The Russian woman is flesh and blood, nerves and temperament, has heart, brain, body and mind where the English girl is flat and nude as a face painted on a playing card; she is without depth, without range, without intricacy. (53-54)

These two characters, Ford's Annabella and Tolstoy's Anna, are not just models of two different literary forms or of two different literary periods, but of two different kinds of relations to imaginal others.

When we reviewed Mead's theory of imaginal dialogues we followed the development of thought's interlocutors from the specific persona of childhood play to the generalized other of abstract thought. However if we focus on the development of dramatic thought then our emphasis will be on coming to know the imaginal others in all their specificity.

In this instance, a high degree of articulation of the imaginal other as well as a multiplicity of figures will characterize development. The more detailed the characterization of the other, the more differentiated is the characterization of the self. Novelists and playwrights are excellent guides in this domain. Many, such as Elizabeth Bowen, speak of patiently placing themselves in the presence of the imaginal other, and observing the details of the other's being. "They reveal themselves slowly to the novelist's perception—as might fellow-travellers seated opposite in a dimly-lit railway carriage" (1975, 172).

Trollope, writing in 1833, described how, in order to make his readers intimately acquainted with his characters, he himself had to get to know each figure in great detail.

> ...and [the author] can never know them well unless he can live with them in the full reality of established intimacy. They must be with him as he lies down to sleep, and as he wakes from his dreams. He must learn to hate them and to love them. He must argue with them, quarrel with them, forgive them, and even submit to them. He must know of them whether they be cold-blooded or passionate, whether true or false, and how far true, and how far false. The depth and the breadth, and the narrowness and the shallowness of each should be clear to him. And as, here in our outer world, we know that men and women

> change—become worse or better as temptation or conscience may guide them—so should these creations of his change, and every change should be noted by him. On the last day of each month recorded, every person in his novel should be a month older than on the first. If the would-be novelist has aptitudes that way, all this will come to him without much struggling;—but if it do not come, I think he can only make novels of wood.
>
> It is so that I have lived with my characters, and thence has come whatever success I have obtained. There is a gallery of them, and of all in that gallery I may say that I know the tone of the voice, and the colour of the hair, every flame of the eye, and the very clothes they wear. Of each man I could assert whether he would have said these or the other words; of every woman, whether she would then have smiled or so have frowned. (1833/1930, 49-50)

The development of depth of characterization corresponds to the development of the character's autonomy. As the character becomes more autonomous, we know about its world not just from external observation or supposition but from the character directly. The author or narrator becomes less omniscient and can be surprised by the other. Observation of the character's actions can be supplemented by the character's own account of thoughts, feelings and wishes through which the imaginal other gains interiority and depth.

In a study of schizophrenics' representations of imaginal figures in dreams, I found that the imaginal other (not the "I" of the dream) was often known only in terms of his/her behavior or action, and not in terms of thoughts, feelings, or wishes (Watkins, 1978). The descriptions of others were neither vivid nor realistic, but shallow and superficial. The dream ego did not respond to the character's feelings and thoughts, thus de-centering the dream ego position, but assimilated the other's actions with respect to the dream ego's feelings and thoughts. Rather than pathology having to do with an over-articulation of an imaginary being and a weak ego or "I," pathology coincided with shallowness in the characterization of the imaginal other and a marked egocentricity in which the imaginal other is known only insofar as it effects the "I." Jung observed in schizophrenia and other forms of dissociation that characters such as homunculi, dwarfs, and boys often appeared having no individual characteristics at all (Jung and Kerenyi, 1949, 84).

Both in acting and in fiction-writing, the actor or writer becomes absorbed in the details of the imaginal other's character, life, and point of view. For Henry James, "the artist is one on whom nothing is lost," and he accused bad authors of "weak specification." But as Flannery O'Connor points out,

> ...to say that fiction proceeds by the use of detail does not mean the simple, mechanical piling up of detail. Detail has to be controlled by some overall purpose, and every detail has to be put to work for you. Art is selective. What is there is essential and creates movement. (1961, 93)

The detailing work of the imaginal realm is not the same as that of the naturalistic realm. In the imaginal work, says O'Connor, details do not seek merely to replicate nature but "while having their essential place in the literal level of the story, operate in depth as well as on the surface" (1961, 71). That is, the selectivity of details contributes to their resonance on a symbolic level. Not all is said about a character but just enough detail. Virginia Woolf says of George Eliot's characters, "even in the least important, there is a roominess and margin where those qualities lurk which she has no call to bring from their obscurity" (1925, 172). All that is presented, however, should be essential: "Every sentence in dialogue should be descriptive of the character who is speaking" (Bower, 1975, 181). The mind that comes to know the character, James said, should be "the most polished of possible mirrors." That is, it should reflect the other rather than using the other as a prop in telling his own story.

Stanislavski, the famous Russian trainer of actors, taught that an actor should "not...present merely the external life of his characters," but create the "inner life of human spirit" (1936, 14).

> A playwright rarely describes the past or the future of his characters, and often omits details of their present life. An actor must complete his character's biography in his mind from beginning to end because knowing how the character grew up, what influenced his behavior, and what he expects his future to be will give more substance to the present life of the character. (Moore, 1974, 30)

Let us look more formally at dimensions that would specify depth of characterization in imaginal dialogues: degree of animation of the imaginal other, degree of articulation of psychological properties, degree of complexity of perspective on the character, and degree of specification of the identity of the character. These dimensions (outlined below) represent movement from a character in an imaginal dialogue who is a passive recipient of the other's actions—without thoughts, feelings, actions, or identity of her own—to a character whose identity is known, whose psychological properties (thoughts, feelings, and wishes) are articulated from both an internal and an external point of view, who is an active agent in her own right, and who is not just a one dimensional, stereotypic figure of only negative or only positive attributes.

1. *Degree of animation*
   a.   Character is passive recipient of other's actions; character does not act or speak. Character is a prop for the other's actions and perceptions.
   b.   Character is again the recipient of the other's actions, but acts or speaks in response to these actions. However character does not initiate actions.
   c.   Character initiates actions and/or dialogue. He or she is no longer a passive recipient and reactive responder. Character can act upon the other(s) present (see Lowe, 1975).

2. *Degree of articulation of psychological properties*
   a.   Character is known by actions alone.
   b.   Psychological properties (thoughts, feelings, and wishes) are attributed to the character by another character or by the self (acting as a kind of narrator). Psychological properties are known from an external point of view only.
   c.   Psychological properties are expressed by the character. They are known from an internal point of view and imply a self-conscious- ness on the part of the character.

As the imaginal other's psychological properties become known from an internal point of view, the imaginal other is further liberated from being but an extension of the ego. Now the imaginal other's motivations, for instance, can be shown to contrast with the ones attributed to him or her by the imaginer.

When a character is known only from its behavior or from an external point of view, the understanding of it is often superficial, fragmented, or distorted. The imaginer often assimilates and reduces the character's actions to the set of meanings which are important to the ego, thus failing to allow the character's presence and point of view to de-center the habitual stance of the ego. The imaginer too quickly assumes she understands what a character wants or feels, without so much as attempting to ask. It is such assumptions that change a basic *telos* of the experience of imagining itself from counteracting egocentricity to sustaining it. In the latter instance the imaginal scene and its people become servants to the usual, most powerful point of view. In the former, as a character's thoughts, feelings, and motivations become known from its own point of view, it is freed from being but a prop to the habitually central voice.

When one has no empathy for the other's point of view his or her actions often become incomprehensible. The members of the self-other dyad are represented as acting either in mutual isolation or else in such a way that the other's action is assimilated to the point of view of the ego. The motive or purpose which organizes various actions into a meaningful pattern is missing. In Burke's terminology (1945), the other, the agent, becomes less differentiated from the scene. Sometimes the motivation is then seen as coming from the outside, from a third party who can control actions from afar. The (imagining) ego is caught not in a world of the other's larger acts, but in the other's series of fragmented behaviors. Action is not organized into complex units, and there is no complex general project to which smaller units of action are subordinated (Watkins, 1978, 54-55).

However the virtue of not knowing from the others' point of view their motivations and thoughts, is that indeed the scene can then be an expression of the imagining ego's point of view. The satisfactions of egocentricity can go undisturbed by a semi-autonomy of the other.

3. *Degree of complexity of perspective on the character*
   a. Character is known from an external perspective only. Although the character may act and may be attributed psychological properties, it is given no voice. The motivations for his or her actions are assumed.
   b. Character is known from an internal perspective. He expresses a point of view. His actions are understood from his point of view only.

c. Character is known from internal and external points of view. Here there is an alternation of perspectives on the character so that his actions and speech can be understood from both his point of view and from the other's. Here one sees and can be seen.

At the beginning of this continuum (a), where the first character is known only through the second's eyes, the first character serves the second's self-image; for example, an assailant is created to sustain the other's role as an innocent victim. At the end of this continuum (c), one character's reality can be challenged by the other. The scene is deepened as the possibility arises for different construals or perspectives. "Characters possess degrees of being in proportion to the variety of perspectives from which they can with justice be perceived" (Burke, 1945, 503).

4. *Degree of specification of identity of character*
   a. The imaginal presence of the other is indicated by the self's speech but by no other indication. The self speaks as thou to someone, but it is not clear to whom.
   b. The imaginal presence of the other can be noted by the linguistic structure of the thought or speech. For instance the phrases of speech meet the constraints of conversation or of dialogue, not monologue: where there is a question, an answer follows; where there is a comment, an acknowledgment follows. This is so despite the absence of any indication that the person is speaking to an imaginal other who has an identity other than that of the habitual self—such as a change in intonation, addressing a character by name or, if in play, designating a different play object to represent a character. Much of thought has this implicitly dialogical structure with no clear articulation as to who the speakers are; i.e., "Now what shall I do today? How about finishing up the paper? I don't think there is enough time. You always say that."

   For instance in the following segment of play, despite the absence of explicit reference to a separate character by name, changes in voice, or gesture, one can detect a conversation going on, an imaginal dialogue, between two voices which can be described as a "supportive instructor" voice and a "pupil" voice.

Example: David is engaged in solitary play with a tinker toy. He says the following: "The wheels go here, the wheels go here. Oh, we need to start it all over again. We need to close it up. See, it closes up. We're starting it all over again. Do you know why we wanted to do that? Because I needed it to go a different way. Isn't it going to be pretty clever, don't you think? But we have to cover up the motor just like a real car." (Kohlberg, *et al.*, 1968, 695)

c. The other presents him or herself as a specific identifiable personality.

CHAPTER TEN

Relativizing the Ego and the Birth of Dialogue

As psychic life is peopled with multiple characters who enjoy varying degrees of autonomy and who are known in their complexity, there occurs a radical shift with respect to the "ego." The "I" becomes not just the one who observes the others. It is now seen as well. It too is like a character, with certain styles of being and interacting which the imaginal others recognize: organizer, narrator, confidant, supervisor. One character may see "ego" as power hungry, another as an infidel, always deserting him or her. Each reveals a different persona, often eclipsing our habitual conceptions of ourselves. As the imaginal others speak and act, they do not just answer the "I's" questions, but speak about the "I" and also about their relations with each other, seemingly apart from the ego. As in literature,

> [the] characters do not develop only single and linear roads of destiny but are, so to speak, human crossroads. It is within this pattern, this meshing together of individualities, that they preserve their autonomy...(Harvey, 1965, 69)

Through this process there is a relative de-centration of psychic life, which can restrict the strength and functions of the ego. Truth becomes redefined. It is not the province of a single voice, but arises between the voices at the interface of the characters' multiple perspectives.

This narrowing of the ego's domain, this view of the ego as another character, would at first seem antithetical to the current trend of ego psychology in the direction of ego strengthening. Hillman

(1975b, 25-26) points out that in psychoanalytic thought a dominant fantasy is the Roman-like process of ego development. Consider Freud's description of this process:

> To strengthen the ego, to make it more independent of the superego, to widen the field of perception and enlarge its organization so that it can appropriate fresh portions of the id, where id was there the ego should be. It is a work of culture. (Freud, 1932/1965, 106)

In a more polycentric psychology, this gradual assimilation of other portions of psyche by the ego is not the goal. In a polycentric psychology, one attuned to and respectful of the multiplicity of the Self, one would attempt to restore some autonomy to the colonies. One function of personifying is "to save the diversity and autonomy of the psyche from dominion by any single power.... Personifying is the soul's answer to egocentricity" (Hillman, 1975b). The ego, though not strengthened through the assimilatory process envisioned by Freud, is nonetheless fortified as its function becomes one of being aware of the multiplicity around and within it.

Not only is there a multiplicity of imaginal others experienced in the distance, but the "I" changes role or identity, as in dreams and playing—now whiny child, now scientist, now sophisticated cosmopolitan. The everyday subtle changes in intonation, gesture, or mood give way to the imaginal figures beneath them, as happens in a dream, where anger may be revealed as a lion or Hitler, or an unknown rapist.

This shift in the position and function of the "I," its relativization, is a primary difference between modern and pre-modern novels. D. H. Lawrence writes that "You mustn't look in my novels for the old stable ego of character. There is another ego, according to whose action the individual is unrecognizable" (1962, 282). Robert Kiely, in a discussion of Lawrence and James Joyce, notices that in their work the "self is released from the prison of 'stable form;' it is projected into the environment, freed to move from shape to shape" (1980, 11). Modern novelists for the most part have abandoned an omniscient narrator who tells the readers the "truth" about each character, who sees the characters as extensions of himself. Now the characters are more often free to tell their own stories, and the tale of each is relativized by the voices of the others.

Luigi Pirandello's play, *Six Characters in Search of an Author*, classically portrays this situation. Here the six characters enter a theater where a play is being rehearsed. They attempt to tell their stories in an effort to find an author who will help let their suffering be known. Each character has his or her own version which pits itself against the others' in an effort to claim reality.

In studying the dramatic nature of thought we need to become familiar with all the modes of narration exhibited in literature. They will help us see how variously we each organize the multiplicity we find within thought—how we, like authors, shift between omniscient and non-omniscient postures with respect to the voices we encounter in dreams, fantasy and thought. In the omniscient novels of the past[26] the author or one of his characters would describe all the other characters in the beginning of the work. The characters' attributed dispositions were then borne out in subsequent scenes. The belief among novelists of this period (from Trollope through Austen) appears to have been that an accurate accounting of who one is can either be given as a static description of characteristics or a listing of how one responds externally to a series of situations (Daiches, 1960, 15).

The critic David Daiches points out that in the nineteenth-century novel

> characters were deployed before the reader (author and reader standing together, as it were, on the reviewing stand, with the author where necessary whispering explanatory remarks into the reader's ear) and revealed their inward development by their outward behavior. The correlation between internal and external, between moral or intellectual development and appropriate observable action or in-action was taken for granted. (1960, 2)

Standing there together amidst a stable hierarchical society, the author could take it for granted that he and the reader shared the same sense

---

[26] As we shall see in Chapter Eleven, the novel was born during a historical period when the experience of hearing voices was being turned over by religion to psychiatry. It is little wonder, then, that the surrender and devotion to voices so characteristic of the religious experience should be carefully avoided by the early novelists, who seemed to control the medley of characters mediated by the novel much as God had his creatures. Paradoxically, during the Romantic period, as religion continued to lose to science its dominion over the definition of reality, literature began to assume some of the functions of religion *vis a vis* respect for the autonomy of the voices.

of what was significant in life. "What was significant in human events was itself manifested in publicly visible doing or suffering, in action or passion related to status or fortune" (Daiches, 1960, 4). Omniscient narration was possible because people agreed about the nature and perception of reality. Reality was something objective, something "out there."

Just as astronomy had displaced man from the center so had philosophy, and so would literature in its turn. Locke argued that we each know our own impressions of reality but not reality *per se*. If reality itself is not knowable, what happens to a literature "whose object is the imitation of reality? It too is then destined to undergo a shift of center" (Tuveson, 1974, 25-26).

It was not simply that omniscience began to fade as one narrative technique replaced another. But rather the omniscient style became an impossibility for many authors, partly because reality itself seemed to be changing. It changed as the twentieth century approached, bringing with it the horrors of world wars, the thriving of multiple and discrepant ideologies, and the insights of a new science, and psychology. The objective position became untenable, leaving us to see how we each effect the known. Nowadays we might nostalgically side with Virginia Woolf in looking back on Jane Austen's period when the world was a commonly shared one. Woolf remarks of Austen:

> To believe that your impressions hold good for others is to be released from the cramp and confinement of personality. One of the marks of the modern novelist is that he is unable to hold that belief. (quoted in Daiches, 1960, 3)

And thus the author had to find a different place to stand in relation to the characters.

Modern literary criticism is filled with debates about what happens when the previously omniscient author withdraws from the work and allows the characters to carry the drama (see Harvey, 1965). Even if the characters appear spontaneously and have their own ideas about the unfolding drama, does not the author observe and coordinate these events, searching for the most expressive details and moments to convey the plot?

In short in imaginal dialogues in which the ego is made relative and non-omniscient, it does not cease to fulfill important functions. A part of the ego—sometimes called the "observing ego"—sometimes the "reflective self-representation" (Schafer, 1968)—is an agent for an awareness of the dialogue as it unfolds. We can liken this part of the Self to a stage manager, narrator, or "histor,"[27] or to the internal observer that actors become aware of when they are playing a part. In Stanislavski's words,

> As I was taking my bath I recalled the fact that while I was playing the part of the Critic I still did not lose the sense of being myself... Actually, I was my own observer at the same time that another part of me was being a fault-finding, critical creature... I divided myself, as it were, into two personalities. One continued as an actor, the other was an observer. Strangely enough this duality not only did not impede, it actually promoted my creative work.
>
> An actor is split into two parts when he is acting. You recall how Tommaso Salvini put it: "An actor lives, weeps and laughs, he observes his own tears and mirth. It is this double existence, this balance between life and acting that makes for art."
>
> As you see, this division does no harm to inspiration. On the contrary the one encourages the other. Moreover we lead a double existence in our actual lives. But this does not prevent our living and having strong emotions. (1936, 19, 167)

This division is like the one we experience when we read and imagine. The book's scene is more vivid to us than the one we literally inhabit—as is the imaginal other with whom we converse in thought. But at the same time there exists ready to hand what Schumaker calls "aesthetic distance," the realization that the imaginal scene exists in a universe apart from the room we are literally in. Some portion of awareness stands ready to see both realities (Schumaker, 1960, 15).

Schafer speaks of this process in psychoanalytic terms, maintaining that what differentiates daydreams from psychosis is the presence or easy recall of a "reflective self representation," that is, an "implicit or explicit notation accompanying realistic thought that it is thought

---

[27] The "histor" seeks to "find out the truth from the various" characters. He is "the narrator as inquirer, constructing a narrative on the basis of such evidence as he has been able to accumulate. The 'histor' is not a character in the narrative, but he is not exactly the author himself either. He is a persona, a projection of the author's empirical virtues" (Scholes and Kellogg, 1966, 262, 265*ff*).

(e.g., memory, perception, anticipation, etc.) and not concrete reality" (1968, 109). In a fantasy which revolves around an imaginal figure, there is a "splitting of the ego" which "allows other ego processes to remain realistically oriented to internal and external circumstances and to note the actual absence of the imagined person..." (Schafer, 1968, 111). Whereas, in psychosis, there is a "limited or slow reversibility of the suspension of the reflective self representations" that occur in daydreams (96).

To enrich our thinking about these changes in "reflective self representation" and "the ego," let us return to literature and see how it dealt with the deterioration of the omniscient stance—again analogizing the author and "her" characters to ego and "its" multiplicity. The decline of the omniscient narrator in fiction—often it was the author's voice—did not entail the end of narrators. Rather narrators joined the ranks of characters. They too became fallible, their perspectives assailable.

What kind of narrators succeeded in carrying on within this more complicated reality? Might these narrators not be models for an ego struggling amidst the multiplicity of mind? Let us look briefly to those employed by Flaubert, James, and Conrad.

Flaubert tried consciously to remove himself from the narrative in *Madame Bovary* and found "that if the omniscient author is eliminated, the only remaining basis for the 'point of view' that justifies the text has to be the consciousness of someone: a character of the novel" (Morrisette, 1961-62, 4). With a decline in omniscience there was a heightened sensitivity to character. Flaubert became so involved in the process of transition from one character's point of view to another that he suggested "that a novel could be written whose value would lie not in its subject at all but in its relationships and articulations: *un livre sur rien*, a book about nothing" (Morrisette, 1961-62, 4). Here Flaubert came close to that aspect of imagination that is based not on story or plot but on the relationship between characters, between points of view. It is the ongoing, ever evolving imagination that does not cease with this denouement or that chapter. Flaubert conceived of a novel more like the conversations in thought (a novel later to be written by Nathalie Saurraute and James Joyce, among others). It has been said of the works of Joyce and Faulkner that such a novel becomes an existence in itself—it is not about something, it is something (Szanto, 1972, 5).

Henry James also realized that surrendering the omniscient stance meant that he must discover some other center or focus through which the story could be told. To achieve this the author must leave himself and enter the consciousness of the character: "A beautiful infatuation this, always, I think, the intensity of the creative effort to get into the skin of the creature" or character (James, quoted in Friedman, 1955, 1161).

But through what kind of consciousness should the story be seen? James felt this character should be "finely aware," "an illuminating intelligence," his mind a "lucid reflector" and "the most polished of possible mirrors." The new narrator must not only have the capacity to be agitated by what he sees. He must also have the capacity to be surprised, even bewildered. Edith Wharton agreed with James:

> It should be the storyteller's first care to choose his reflecting mind deliberately, as one would choose a building site...and when this is done, to live inside the mind chosen, trying to feel, see and react exactly as the latter would, no more, no less and, above all, no otherwise. Only thus can the writer avoid attributing incongruities of thought and metaphor to his chosen interpreter. (quoted in Friedman, 1955, 1165)

The author gradually receded from the novel. He intruded less and in some cases disappeared altogether. James Joyce said that the author was "refined out of existence." As Friedman (1955) points out, this refinement entailed gradually limiting the author's channels of information and possible vantage points by staying within the consciousness of a particular character or set of characters.

This limitation of the author's vision—from omniscience to the point of view of a character—reflected a radical change in the function of fiction. Fiction could no longer imitate factual reality, but could only present imaginative reality (Scholes and Kellogg, 1966, 262), that reality to which one has access only through the eyes of characters. In some cases the author handed over his job to a "witness-narrator." Such a character did not possess the omniscience of the author, but through certain devices was able to supplement a merely human understanding of the minds and goings on about him. For example, Joseph Conrad would often use as his narrator a character "in whom others felt compelled to confide," a sharer of secrets. The diaries and letters of others would fall into his possession. It was his or her presence which would be sought by the other characters for their late-night confessionals—in the jungle, by the fire, and at the pub.

Would not such a narrator be a fitting hermetic go-between to the multiple voices one encounters: now a diplomat, now a confidant, now a drinking partner, depending on which character one is trying to understand? The flexibility, intelligence, empathy and savvy required by this kind of ego would be learned by interaction with characters, just as our ease with other people is gained slowly through early bungling, embarrassment, faux pas, and self-centeredness brought "rudely" to our attention.

The development we have been describing does not have to do with the enlargement of the ego or with the building of ego strength in all its aspects. It does however, have to do with an increased ability to allow other voices to speak (which relativizes the ego) and with the increased agility of an observing ego which can be attentive to these imaginal dialogues. This quality of ego which is akin to a narrator cannot be assumed to be present. The ego all too often identifies with a given character without awareness of having done so. For example, take a man who identifies with a strong, independent, masterful character and is unaware that this is but one psychic possibility among many. Though he may alternate between positions of independence and dependence, feelings of strength and feelings of impotence, there may be little or no recognition on his part of these shifts in character.

As imaginal dialogues develop from dialogues in which the "I" is omniscient to ones in which the "I" is one voice among others, the term "dialogue" deepens in meaning. It pertains not only to the linguistic structure of communication between two or more parties, but to that kind of relating—often felt as spiritual—which preserves the integrity of both self and other. One neither abdicates selfhood nor incorporates the other. Each can address and be addressed. The development of this manner of relating—from "I-It" to "I-Thou" relation—is the central theme of Martin Buber's philosophical and religious work.

For Buber these styles of relating are not limited to person-God or person-person relations, but include man's relation to nature and intelligible forms—ideas, deeds, works of art (Pfuetze, 1973, 157). Buber contrasts abstract monologic thinking to dramatic speech-

RELATIVIZING THE EGO

thinking. He finds dialogic thought to be characterized by directedness to an other and openness to the unpredictable: "One can never know what the other will say, nor rehearse one's reply" (Pfuetze, 1973, 129).

In "I-It" relations the other is a thing which I use, experience, or manipulate. I notice only those aspects of him, her, or it which relate to my purpose. I do not come to know the other in her essence. Nor do I come to know more deeply my own being. For Buber each person has two "I's:" the "I" of "I-It" and the "I" of "I-Thou." In "I- It," I am never wholly myself, just as the other is not wholly himself or herself: "I become through my relation to the Thou, as I become I, I say Thou" (Buber, 1958, 11). This development from "I-It" to "I-Thou" is never completed once and for all. One continually falls back into, and then struggles out of, a relation of "I-It."

In *Daniel* Buber (1915) writes that although we may first address the other, eventually we must be able to be addressed by the other—a process analogous to the doll's change from being a passive recipient of the child's action to its increasing animation in early childhood play. It is in this addressing and being addressed in relationship that self-knowledge arises.

Buber argues for a mysticism in which the integrity of both self and other is preserved. He argues against either a dissolution of the self into otherness, or the negation of otherness through the assertion of "the all embracing character of the self" (Pfuetze, 1973, 138). In dialogue one asserts the primacy of relation and struggles to maintain that tension rather than totally identifying with or incorporating the other. Buber firmly asserts the autonomy of the other, working against a theory of imagination that returns all images to the "I."

> The tree is no impression, no play of my imagination, no value depending on my mood; but it is bodied over against me and has to do with me, as I with it—only in a different way. (1958, 8)

Similarly with artistic forms:

> This is the eternal source of art: a man is faced by a form which desires to be made through him into a work. This form is no offspring of his soul, but is an appearance which steps up to it and demands of it the effective power. The man is concerned with an act of his being. If he carries it through, if he speaks the primary word out of

> his being to the form which appears, then the effective power streams out, and the work arises.
>
> I do not behold [the form] as a thing among the "inner" things nor as an image of my "fancy," but as that which exists in the present. If test is made of its objectivity the form is certainly not "there." Yet what is actually so much present as it is? And the relation in which I stand to it is real, for it affects me, as I affect it. (9-10)

The autonomy of the other does not exclude the possibility of putting one's own life into it for a while. Within dialogue there are moments in which one feels as though one were the other. Buber describes being with a pine tree and identifying so completely with the tree that he felt its bark as his own skin and its cones as his own children (1915, 133). In this moment, however, the being of the tree is not reduced to the being of the man. This momentary identification with the tree is similar to Cary's emphasis on the author's sympathy for his character. Dostoevsky, Cary claims, was Ivan while writing "Pro and Contra." Through this sympathy he experienced Ivan's arguments from the inside, even though they contradicted his intentions as author.

For Buber then, true dialogue with an imaginal other is a reciprocal, mutual relation in which the other is autonomous and has the freedom to address as well as to be addressed. In such a dialogue one would approach the other without intending to use or even to "experience" him or her. For in experiencing, Buber claims, we construe that experience arises from a self rather than between oneself and the world: "The world has no part in the experience. It permits itself to be experienced but has no concern in the matter. For it does nothing to the experience, and the experience does nothing to it" (1958, 5). True dialogic relation is not based on verbal exchange, but rather on the autonomy of the other and one's openness to the other. Indeed, there need be no words spoken for such a relation to exist. Though this meeting occasions the development of the "I," it radically mitigates against egocentricity. As dialogue may appear in silence, so may monologue be present within dialogue with another. While all the linguistic requirements of dialogue may be satisfied in a conversation, a relation more akin to monologue, to "I-It" relation, may nonetheless prevail.

For Buber as for Jung, the development of a sense of the other's autonomy does not entail the self's subservience to the other's will; one does not necessarily do what a voice might say. Instead, the autonomy of both sides of the relation—"I" and "Thou"—is retained.

"I-It" and "I-Thou" are two modes of existence which characterize our relationship to others, both literal and imaginal. They correspond to Erich Fromm's distinction between "having" and "being:" "In the having mode of existence my relationship to the world is one of possessing and owning, one in which I want to make everybody and everything including myself, my property" (1976, 12). In the being mode the other is not incorporated and is allowed to change. The other is permitted to exist in his/her autonomy, authenticity, truth, and aliveness. Fromm, in *To Have or To Be*, traces the transition from a societal emphasis on "being" to one on "having," and sees the rise of industrialism as a cultural turning point.

Industrialism, Fromm maintains, succeeded by virtue of two psychological premises:

> (1) that the aim of life is happiness, that is, maximum pleasure, defined as the satisfaction of any desire or subjective need a person may feel (radical hedonism); (2) that egotism, selfishness, and greed, as the system needs to generate them in order to function, lead to peace and harmony. (1976, xxv)

Profit, meanwhile, lost its original meaning of "profit for the soul" and began to mean only material profit.

It may seem farfetched at first to speculate on how these dominant themes—which sustain our present culture, and in part breed our psychologies of imagination—impinge on our relation to imaginal others. However if we look at this transition as it unfolded for the Romantics, we find that while imagination was first lauded for its "sympathy"—its capacity to free us from a self-centered world and allow us into the roles of others—this same chameleon-like activity of imagination was later used to expand the limits of the Self, to enrich the Self with the bounty of the world. The poet would take on the qualities of the other—literal or imaginal—in order to expand himself. The rhetoric and sales pitches of much contemporary popular psychology concerning the imagination reflects this shift. We are urged to "expand our potential" through tapes and exercises that treat the figures of the imaginal like consumer merchandise, like pawns of the ego to be used only for its own enrichment and betterment. In therapy where imaginal dialogues can be observed in detail, one often finds the characters themselves objecting to being treated as the ego's objects: being used, being lectured to, being "had."

In noting these differences among imaginal dialogues, we are moving toward considerations of pathology. Though we have argued against many of the usual notions of pathology with regard to the imaginal we can now begin, from a standpoint of basic respect for the imaginal, to articulate how the viewpoint presented here might itself conceive of development and pathology.

PART IV

*Therapeutic Implications:
Entertaining Voices*

CHAPTER ELEVEN

The Voices of Hallucination

By now it should be clear that it has been our modern scientific conceptions of reason and reality—and the social conventions that result from them—that have dictated our psychological theories of imaginal dialogues. These same conceptions are responsible for assigning pathology and devising treatment strategies. It should come as no surprise that the brand of imaginal dialogues commonly referred to as "hearing voices" or "hallucination" should have fallen prey to historical shifts toward secular and scientific conceptions of reason and reality—shifts which have led our society to laud imageless logic as the very apex of reason and thought and to promote the perceptible as the only legitimate reality.

Imaginal dialogues are often looked at askance by clinicians. The suggestion that a person ought to entertain more characters, allow them greater autonomy, and enable characterizations to unfold which are more vivid and articulated might lead many to believe that we are encouraging hallucination, dissociation or fragmentation of the personality, a dangerous weakening of the ego—and perhaps even that we recommend becoming a "split personality."

However as we have seen, the entertaining of a multiplicity of autonomous and vivid characters is commonplace in the creation of literature and the practice of religion, and is hardly synonymous with pathology. The term "hearing voices" immediately warns us of the monological and non-reciprocal nature of many of these experiences where one receives, hears, the voice's message but does not necessarily respond to the voice or engage it in dialogue. It also warns us of the often undeveloped nature of the characters involved, as it is often just the voice that comes to be known.

What a culture designates as psychopathological reflects its values and assumptions, its goals for thought and behavior. We can see this when we examine "hallucinations." *The Oxford English Dictionary* (1933) reveals that the word is relatively new, having entered the English language in 1646 with the Enlightenment, and only gaining its present meaning in the last century with the births of psychiatry and psychology as sciences.[28] As a word it is derived from the Latin *(h)allucinari*; to wander in mind, to talk idly. Its first meanings (in 1652) were "to be deceived, suffer illusion, entertain false notions, blunder, mistake" (*Compact Edition of the Oxford English Dictionary,* 1971, 1245). In the nineteenth century it took on its modern meaning of an apparent perception which lacks an object (*Larger Oxford English Dictionary*, 1933, 44). The gist of the earlier definition—to mistake, to entertain false notions, to blunder—was certainly carried forward and helped allocate hallucinations to the bins of psychopathology. Gradually the definitions of "delusion," "hallucination," and "illusion" were again differentiated.[29] The presence of hallucinations in persons not suffering from drug toxicity, neurological difficulties or fever was taken as a symptom of schizophrenia.

Where had hallucinations been in Western conceptions before the nineteenth century? Certainly the experience of what is now called "hallucination" was not an altogether new movement of mind. Before the rise of science with its focus on objectivity, and the secularization of experience, what are now designated as hallucinations, were probably thought of as visions: "The action or fact of seeing or contemplating something not actually present to the eye;" "something which is apparently seen otherwise than by ordinary sight; especially

---

[28] Sarbin and Juhasz (1967, 1) note the first English use of the word hallucination in a translation of Lavater's *Of Ghostes and Spirites Walking by Nyght* in 1572. In this work hallucinations were "ghostes and spirites walking by nyght, and strange noyses, crackes, and sundry forwarnynges, whiche commonly happen before the death of menne, great slaughters and alterations of kyngdomes."

[29] Van den Berg (1982a) notes that Asclepiades made use of historical sources to differentiate between hallucinations and illusions, and that the Asclepian differentiation between these phenomena is much like our modern notions. Despite this early treatment, however, English definitions did not distinguish these phenomena until Esquirol's work (1833, 1838) became widely known.

an appearance of a prophetic or mystical character, or having the nature of a revelation, supernaturally presented to the mind in sleep or in an abnormal state" (*Shorter Oxford English Dictionary*, 1933, 2363).

While many visions were valued as means of access to God and His angels, to the Virgin Mary and other saints, other visions were dealt with as blunders. As remote as psychiatry's current notions of hallucination may seem from the earlier treatment of visions by the Church and its Inquisitors, the former derives in part from the latter.

Sarbin and Juhasz have traced the curious history of how the mystic and Scholastic treatments of visions became assimilated into the medical model of hallucination. Just as the psychiatrist must distinguish between "ordinary" imaginal experience and "hallucination," so did the early Church fathers distinguish between various kinds of visions. The mystics' treatment of vision is exemplified by St. Augustine (1967, 354-430), who diagnosed how far removed the vision was from immediate sense experience. He judged it superior the more intellectualized and immaterial it was (as with a Platonic idea) and the further removed from the sounds of time, space, and corporeality. The Scholastics, exemplified by St. Thomas Aquinas (1225-1274), diagnosed visions not in terms of level of embodiment (corporeal versus intellectual or immaterial), but in terms of the source and content of imaginary experience. While visions were valued as bridges between man and the supernatural, the region of the supernatural with which one was in contact was of the greatest concern. St. Thomas and his followers had the difficult task of determining whether the source of the vision was celestial, infernal or natural—whether the figures were those aligned with God or those with the Devil.[30] Their task was further complicated by the fact that the Devil was known to tell falsehoods and to disguise himself in the costumes of those closest to God. Fortunately the Devil was more likely to appear corporeally than intellectually. But the question of level could not definitively differentiate between visions. Those visionaries entertaining figures from

---

[30] The psychoanalyst Leston Havens (1981) has proposed that the difference between saints and hallucinating patients may have to do with the kind or quality of advice the voice or figure gives the patient. This is a kind of differentiation based on what the voices have to say, rather than whether they are perceptual or non-perceptual. It is thus analogous to the older differentiation between the interlocutors, the "who's," of imaginal dialogues. Development in this model is described as "upgrading" the voices who give bad advice, by voices gradually becoming more like the analyst's voice.

non-Christian mythology were publicly derided, humiliated, and sometimes burned at the stake as witches along with those who were considered "demoniacal or out of their senses or if the source of their vision appeared Satanic" (Sarbin and Juhasz, 1967, 341).

St. Ignatius (1491-1556) also concerned himself with the source of the vision and created a precedent for *ex post facto* analysis of hallucination later to be borrowed by psychiatry: if the effect of the vision is good, it is from God; if it is bad, it is from the Devil (Sarbin and Juhasz, 1967, 342). The modern version goes as follows: if the person is considered insane, the imagining is thought of as a hallucination and as bad; if the person is considered of sound mind, the imagining is either creative or strange, but not bad.

St. Theresa of Avila (1515-1582) is given the critical role of being the first religious figure to favor turning over to medicine the diagnosis of visions and imaginings. To protect her visionary nuns from the purges of the Inquisition, she argued "that certain imaginings may be the effect of infirmities and sickness and, as such, persons experiencing them were not responsible" (Sarbin and Juhasz, 1967, 343). Natural sources such as melancholy, a weak imagination, drowsiness, and sleep or sleep-like states were seen to vie with celestial and infernal sources, thus liberating the seer from a negative diagnosis of demon dealings.

While saving visions from the Devil—and thus the visionary from the stake—this reassessment also caused visions to begin to lose their positive association with God and the angels. The visionary and her visions were delivered to the asylum, and there the doctor was given the task of diagnosing the reported imaginings of the patient. He already knew certain facts about the imaginer—that others suspected the patient of insanity, had observed what they considered inappropriate behavior (particularly inappropriate role behavior), and had found the patient disturbing to be around. The doctor needed these other facts to formulate a diagnosis:

> The choice of words and the syntactical arrangement are not sufficient criteria for the diagnoser to make a confident judgment of hallucination unless he is willing to run the risk of mislabelling the imaginal and verbal products of poets and playwrights and nearly everybody else. Since spoken or written reports may obscure truth through ellipsis and metaphor, the diagnoser has no

choice but to use as his raw data observations other than the spoken or written reports of imaginings. These other observations focus on the psychological status conferred on the suspected hallucinatory concurrent with his other statuses, such as mental hospital patient, poet, novelist, etc. (Sarbin, 1967, 374)

The medicalization of the societal approach to imagining was unfortunate for a number of reasons. While St. Theresa had argued that it was "as if," her sisters were ill, medicine dropped the "as if," turning metaphor into fact. This "fact" then called for doctors to devise treatments for the imaginings that had always existed. Though the hallucination was no longer labeled in terms of level (higher or lower), content, or source (celestial or infernal), the hallucinator was labeled insane or sick (Sarbin and Juhasz, 1967).

Rather than discriminate between voices the physician needed only to discriminate between image and "reality" to determine whether or not the reported imaginings were erroneous.

> This judgment, just as in the case of the Augustinian practitioner, was a rather complex inference requiring great language sophistication and a large number of shared concepts on the part of the both speaker and hearer. However, because of the new pseudo-objective terminology, the practitioner probably considered the judgment to be a simple, scientific diagnosis. For example, a memory-image of a picture of the Virgin that the subject had seen before would not have been an erroneous image. On the other hand, the image (memory-image) of the village washerwoman, if called "The Virgin Mary" by the seer would have constituted an erroneous image. By the scientific rules of the time, the image of any mythological figure, if taken for "reality" would have constituted an erroneous image. The physician was thus called upon to distinguish between the various senses of identical words: Whether they were meant literally ["I (corporeally) now see the Virgin Mary"] or figuratively ["(It is as if) I now see the Virgin Mary"]. (Sarbin and Juhasz, 1967, 345-346)

The doctor's job was to judge the imaginings of people already considered insane. The presence of hallucinations was a criterion for being insane, but a patient's presumed insanity predisposed the doctor to judge his imaginings as hallucinations—a diagnosis derived from circular reasoning.

Esquirol's (1833, 1838) work set the stage for the consolidation of the medical model of hallucination. He distinguished illusions from hallucinations and argued that while illusions may appear in healthy people, hallucinations are invariably pathological. This meant that despite people's commitment to systems of reality different from that of modern science, their visions, in retrospect, could be diagnosed as crazy. Socrates, St. Catherine of Siena, Dante, and countless others now became victims of the medicalization of imagination.

In the late 1800s the new psychologists in their treatment of hallucination, looked back to such experiences as the inner voice Socrates relied upon to admonish him when doing something undesirable to a god, the being who followed Descartes down streets urging him not to abandon his search for truth, to Swedenborg's conversations with angelic visitors, and to Saint Catherine's espousal to Christ and called these all hallucinations, "fallacies of perception" (Parish, 1897, 39, 77-78). The possible desirability of such experiences was rarely acknowledged as the emphasis was on differentiating the perceptual from the imaginal, on establishing the claim that such experiences are internal and psychological rather than external and "real." Rather than searching for distinctions between various imaginal experiences, the focus was on differentiating the "purely" perceptual from the imaginal.

The psychologists who took part in this movement began to meet with protest beginning in the middle of the last century and continuing into the present century (Michea, 1846; Brierre de Boismont, 1859; Ball, 1883; Gurney and Myers, 1884; William James, 1892). But the protest was interrupted by World War I and its message faded away as behaviorism displaced the study of consciousness, thought, and imagery (Sarbin and Juhasz, 1967, 352). An interesting opposition to the equation of hallucination with pathology emerged at the International Congress of Psychology in Paris in 1889. Psychologists such as Sidgewick protested that hallucinations occurred not just in persons of "morbid" personality but in perfectly healthy people as well and proposed a census (The International Census of Waking Hallucinations in the Sane) to prove it. In 1894 Sidgewick studied 15,316 people of good health, who had not suffered from mental illness. He found that 7.8 percent of the 7717 men and 12 percent of the 7599 women reported having hallucinatory experiences. Given the prevalent equation of severe mental illness with the occurrence of hallucination, it would not be surprising if the actual percentage were even higher due to people's fears of admitting to such experience. The census, however, did not successfully dissolve the equation between hallucination and mental illness. Before this equation could be challenged psychology's commitment to a scientifically defined notion of reality would have to be addressed.

On close inspection of examples of hallucination in the psychiatric literature, one finds that the term "hallucination" is a general category for a broad array of experiences. In all instances it is a pejorative term. For example, hallucinations can be experienced through all the sensory modes. They can be experienced as occurring inside or outside the body, confused with the perceptual or merely experienced alongside the perceptual, or fleeting impressions or almost continuous presences. Fundamental to the various theories, however, is the notion of the perceptual or quasi-perceptual nature of hallucinations and, correspondingly, their appearance in "normal" space, be that inside or outside the physical body. Here we confine our interest to hallucinations which involve an imaginal figure, although our critique of the treatment of these kinds of hallucinations in the literature will have more general implications for other forms of hallucination as well.

The emphasis in theories of hallucination lies predominantly on the following two commitments and priorities: 1) that which arises from perception and sensation should be more vivid than that which arises from imagination;[31] the objective world, the consensually agreed upon, should be more vivid than the imaginal and the subjective; 2) external space should be reserved for perceptual and objectively verifiable phenomena. Thus the imaginal, which is subjective, should be experienced in internal "psychological" space. When these rules are broken—when an imaginal figure appears perceptually and externally, or rivals the perceptual in intensity—the resulting experience is labeled a hallucination. The hallucination breaks in upon the usual vision of reality. Pathology becomes coincident with a failure to experience images as internal and/or a preoccupation with imaginal persons or events that rival the perceptual in intensity or compromise its agreed-upon priority. When one experiences an event

---

[31] Sarbin points out that commitment to the assertion that perception and sensation should be radically distinguishable from the imaginal was falsified over a century ago by Galton and by the classic experiments of Seashore in 1895, Perky in 1910, and Wilson in 1941. In these experiments images and percepts are confused by normal subjects "under conditions of poor illumination and sound or in ecological settings that are impoverished for familiar cues" (Sarbin, 1967, 377).

which breaks through the usual conventions concerning the internal and the external, the imaginary and the perceptual, one can "feel" crazy or fear craziness. Hallucinations most threaten those who conceive of themselves as "in control" (by virtue of their obedience to the perceptual).

The usual psychiatric approach to hallucination is one of efficient cause. The hallucinator, as a result of his "inability to discriminate between thoughts and perceptual experience" (Freeman, Cameron, and McGhie, 1966) or his "failure to maintain an adequate differentiation between internal experiences and the perception of experiences occurring outside the self" (Blatt and Wild, 1967, 18), confuses an internal thought with the objects occurring in ordinary perceptual space. Thus hallucination becomes defined as "an internal image that seems as real, vivid, and external as the perception of an object" (Horowitz, 1970, 8).

The usual therapeutic strategy is to "help" the patient return to the usual notions and values about reality agreed upon in our psychology: namely, that what is not consensually validated should be experienced as internal, residing in psychic space; that this internal experience should not compete with or impair relations to "real" others; that the proper contents of this internal space are not figures but thoughts. An example of this kind of approach to hallucinations is given in Leston Havens' psychoanalytic paper "The placement and movement of hallucinations in space: Phenomenology and theory" (1962). Here a developmental line proposed for hallucinations is a gradual movement of the hallucinated presence from outside the self to inside the self, and ultimately to becoming integrated into the self.

From Havens' point of view the hallucinated figure is experienced in external space in order to satisfy specific needs for external objects (i.e., people). Havens speculates that in some cases the person, because of a failure of introjection, needs an external figure to compensate for the absence of an internal one. For Havens the more "mature position" for the imaginal object is "the position closer to identification" (1962, 432). Thus hallucination becomes defined as "the substitution of an imaginary object for a real one that was never identified with" (434). The rule of thumb is summarized by Jaynes: "When the illness is most severe, the voices are loudest and come from outside; when least severe, voices often tend to be internal whispers; and when internally localized, their auditory qualities are sometimes vague" (1976, 91).

Some phenomenologists (Merleau-Ponty, 1962, 334*ff* and van den Berg, 1982a) have disputed whether the "hallucinator" actually cannot discriminate between a perceptual experience and a hallucinogenic one. Although their examples and arguments do not disprove the existence of such a lack of discrimination, their work introduces differentiation into the less than subtle "perception vs. fallacies of perception" distinction. If one looks closely at first-person accounts of hallucinations, one finds accounts where the patient does not confuse the imaginal voice or figure with his or her perceptions. In *The Autobiography of a Schizophrenic Girl* (Sechehaye, 1951) many such examples are given by the patient, Renee:

> ...strident noises, piercing cries began to hammer in my head. Their unexpectedness made me jump. Nonetheless, I did not hear them as I heard real cries uttered by real people. The noises, localized on the right side, drove me to stop up my ears. But I readily distinguished them from the noises of reality. I heard them without hearing them, and recognized that they arose within me.
>
> I threw things to the right, toward the locked French windows where I localized my Persecutor, the System, Antipiol—pillows, the water pitcher, my comb. I wanted to chase Antipiol, to crush him so that I would no longer hear his voice.
>
> Actually in all honesty, I saw no one. I heard no voice. Yet there it was, not an emptiness, not a silence. There was a considerable difference between this part of the room and the others. The corner at the right was alive, personalized; there was someone very real there, empty though it was.
>
> I continued to respond to voices which, though I actually did not hear them, existed nonetheless for me.
>
> After I left the hospital I no longer heard Antipiol's voice. I say "heard" for I do not know what other word to use to convey the impression of actually hearing an invisible something occupying a corner of the room and saying disagreeable things to which I was obliged to answer. Just the same, I did not really hear them. (42, 62-64)

In these examples the hallucinated figure occurs alongside or amidst[32] perceived objects but is not seen as the same. Such examples allow us to differentiate experiences where the imaginal is confused with the perceptual and those where it is differentiated from the perceptual but granted an equal or greater priority to objective thought and reality. That these two kinds of experience are so rarely differentiated in the literature on hallucination—examples of the latter being identified as the former—points to a failure not just on the patients' parts but on the doctors'; a cultural failure to which doctor and patient are prone in different ways. Hallucinating people do not ask us to come and see the figure, to listen for his words. They are aware that this spectacle, this voice, is in their world and not in the one we share (van den Berg, 1982b). They create special names for these voices and their conversations, differentiating them from those we share: "language magic," "secret language," "painful long-distance conversation," "cold castigation language," "court-of-law punishment language," "deadly language," "grand onanism concert" (Gruhle, 1929). By this language, they make clear to us that the disturbing features of these imaginal experiences lie in the quality of relationship between themselves and the figures—the abusive, cold, distant, judging, deathly forms of being together. When hallucinations are scrupulously imitated by the doctor, and the patient given the task of differentiating this perceptual experience from the hallucinatory one, all non-delirious patients are able to tell the difference (Zucker, 1928).

Our cultural failure is a failure to identify a realm of experience which is not hallucinatory in the strict sense of a confusion with perception, but whose images rival or supplant the priority given to the objective. When this realm is active, a person

> ...does not see and hear in the normal sense, but makes use of his sensory fields and his natural insertion into a world in order to build up, out of the fragments of this world, an artificial world answering to the total intention of his being. (Merleau-Ponty, 1962, 341)

When this intention is given attention the interruptive nature of such experiences—interruptive to the priority of interpersonal and

---

[32] Van den Berg (1982b) emphasizes this quality of the imagining being amidst the perceptual: "Hallucinating, according to its nature, is to see (hear, etc.) that which another does not see, amid that which everyone, including the patient himself, sees. This 'amid' is a prerequisite in the same way as light is a prerequisite of darkness. To hallucinate means to have a world strictly of one's own in the framework of reference in the social world" (160-161).

intersubjective reality—recedes. Too rarely are patients queried closely enough about the nature of their "hallucinatory" experiences to determine whether they are hallucinatory in the strict sense. Such a distinction does not matter to those whose point of view gives unqualified priority to the objective.[33] For instance Havens (1962, 430) describes a woman who experiences her dead father as a constant companion, sitting on her shoulder and talking to her at length. But she does not see him. She knows he is dead, and she comes to know that she should speak to him internally rather than audibly.[34] This experience is more like that of an "imaginary companion" than of a hallucination.

In childhood as in ancient Greece, dreams are experienced as happening in the world—the bedroom, the hall, the closet (Piaget, 1960).

---

[33] Explanations of hallucinations "presuppose the priority of objective thought, and having at their disposal only one mode of being, namely objective being, try to force the phenomenon of hallucination into it. In this way they misconceive it, and overlook its own mode of certainty and its immanent significance since, according to the patient himself, hallucination has no place in objective being" (Merleau-Ponty, 1962, 335).

[34] The person whose imaginings are diagnosed as pathological and/or as "hallucinations" has breached some of the following implicit social contracts (among others) which resulted in having his or her imaginings diagnosed at all: (1) One should either attend to the "real" people present, or pretend to do so (Goffman, 1981). If a person speaks aloud to an imaginal figure in the company of others, he has openly displayed that his attention is elsewhere. (2) One should not request or demand, implicitly or explicitly, that other people attend to one's own inner concerns when one is not attending to these other people (Goffman, 1981). By speaking aloud to an imaginal figure in the company of others, one demands their attention to a reality which is not their own. (3) One should not argue that a world one has access to that others do not equals or exceeds in importance the world that is shared by all. (4) One should not engage in conversation with "imaginary" people when "actual" people are present and presumably willing to converse. (5) When imagining, one should do so internally. One should not experience one's imaginings amidst one's perceptions (i.e., externally). (6) One should ensure that the most vivid experience is intersubjective experience, not private imaginings. Corollary 1: Perception of material reality should always be more vivid than imagining. Corollary 2: Material, secular reality should supplant spiritual reality, if the latter entails entertaining the imaginal figures of a belief system other than the scientific. (7) One should present oneself as unitary. If multiplicity of self is experienced, it should be dealt with through forms of speech that do not challenge a unitary vision of the self (e.g., calling the figures "aspects of myself," "parts of myself," "my personae," "representations of people I have experienced in the past"). (8) One should assume responsibility for one's imaginings: "It is I who create the characters;" "Even though it may seem like she who did it, it was actually I."

In childhood, "The world is still the vague theatre of all experiences" (Merleau-Ponty, 1962, 343). Then the child is taught that his experience is "only a dream:" "Oh, you were only dreaming," says the helpful, reassuring parent, who opens the door of the bedroom closet to show that there is no lion there. "It is just in your mind." The child is taught to withdraw fantasy and dream from the world. When and if it appears there again in adulthood the adult, like the child, becomes terrified; more terrified than the child, not because of the lion but because of the fear of being crazy. What the child is not taught in our culture is that fantasy does sometimes look like perception; how to differentiate the two when they do look alike; how to make it clear to others that one can differentiate between them; and how to treat such experience metaphorically rather than literally. If one can learn these things one is not so pressured to turn one's back on the figures who so clamor to be heard and understood. The patient whose imaginings are subject to the doctor's diagnostic eye must be linguistically sophisticated enough to supply the appropriate qualifiers when under examination: "'It is *as if* I hear a voice,' or 'it *appears* to be a ghost,' or 'I *imagined* I saw the Virgin Mary'" (Sarbin, 1967, 371). When an individual has the linguistic skills necessary to convince the doctor that he is speaking metaphorically but does not use them, the individual is involved in a breach of social contract.

We can approach our preoccupation with hallucination as a by-product of our modern model of mind and reality. Were the imaginal mode more valued in our culture, hallucinations would most likely be seen as visions, as entrances to another, equally or more valued world than the perceptual. The externality, vividness, autonomy, perceptual or quasi-perceptual nature of some imaginal dialogues would not appear problematic. Pathology would have to be redefined in relation to an alternative vision of reality and purpose. Hallucinations signal the power of the imaginal to intrude on ego consciousness. It is a power that is unwelcome to the modern organization and conceptualization of mind, a power that threatens the ego's sense of control and reality.

If we were to adjust our priorities the problematic features of imaginal dialogues would not have to do with their experienced externality, vividness, quasi-perceptual nature, or the autonomy of the figures—as these all contribute to the vivification of an imaginal world—but with those features of some imaginal dialogues that negate or flatten the complexity of each character, making drama superficial and dialogue either impossible or stereotypic. In instances where the imaginal is equated with the perceptual, one would hope to allow it a sense of reality apart from perceptual reality. This is necessary not only for the sake of reality testing but also so that the figures can be heard metaphorically rather than literally. From the viewpoint of valuing the dramatic quality of mind it would not be the quasi-perceptual quality *per se* of an imaginal dialogue that would be worrisome, but the quality of relation between self and imaginal other. It is precisely this focus that Erwin Straus pursues in his classic phenomenological study of hallucinations, "Aesthesiology and Hallucinations."

Hallucinations, says Straus, are pathological variations of the relationship between self and other. In hallucination the relation between self and imaginal other is most often non-reciprocal. The hallucinator feels reached, touched, spoken to by the other—his boundaries are intruded upon—but he cannot reach or touch the other. The self is infinitely reachable, offering no resistance to the other: "[The] patient is denied any spontaneous and free survey of the world; his thoughts being heard, his mind being read, denote that the barriers of his intimate life have been leveled off, that the innermost sphere of his existence has been invaded" (Straus, 1958, 168). Indeed the Self is characterized by a passivity which "removes the reachable to a limitless remoteness" (Straus, 1958, 165). The passivity is often joined by a feeling of impotence.

> The common order of things, in which each object has its place, with its own limited range and sphere of influence, is no longer valid. There are no boundaries...there is no organization of space into danger- and safety-zones. (Straus, 1958, 166)

To reflect, says Straus, one must have a space of detachment in which to stand. While these qualities do not characterize all hallucinations, they are true of a certain class of hallucinations (often associated with schizophrenia and paranoia) in which the imaginal other is an intrusive, condemning, abusive and commanding presence. On inspection it is generally only when the hallucinated imaginal figures take this posture and the hallucinator either responds with acute fear and passivity or takes action in our shared reality to counter the attacks that hospitalization and/or a diagnosis of acute psychosis occurs.[35] The focal feature is not the hallucination's vividness or quasi-perceptual nature, but the nature of the structure of relation between self and imaginal other that is a reflection of that psychical totality which is called pathological.[36] This structure of relation is not specific to imagining and its "hallucinations," but characterizes the person's relation to "actual" others and their other modes of existence.

Straus stresses the annulment of reciprocity between self and other in hallucinatory experiences. The sensory modalities—usually our means of gaining access to the reality of the other—are distorted and inverted. Rather than being our path of access to the richness of the world, it is the hostile other's route to the abnegation of our freedom. Vision is blinded by light rays, by movies projected upon the self. Audition is deafened and defeated by the willful voices of the other. One cannot defend oneself by removing oneself in space or covering one's ears. Touch becomes inverted so that while I cannot touch the other, I am overcome by being sprayed at, blown at, electrified.

The imaginal others turn all their attention on the self. The self feels that all these voices are concerned only with him:

> The *Other* is a realm of the hostile, in which the patient finds himself quite alone and quite defenseless, delivered up to a power that threatens him from all sides. The voices aim at him, they have singled him out, and they separate him from all others. He is certain that they mean him and no other; he is not surprised that his neighbor can hear nothing. Indeed, he is not surprised at all; he does not question, neither himself nor others nor things; he does not test his impressions, nor evaluate them according to general rules. (Straus, 1958, 166)

---

[35] "In my experience hallucinatory objects are most often helpful, approving and loving early in the course of their relationship. The paranoid person is hospitalized only after this friendly period is over and accusations and reproaches have set in" (Havens, 1962, 430).

[36] The Dutch phenomenologist J. H. van den Berg argues, as did Moreau de Tours (1845) earlier, that "A hallucination like any other artificially isolated phenomenon, can only be rightly observed in a study of the psychical totality, which is disturbed in some way. This being-disturbed should be the first and foremost subject of the study. The result of the study can only be called satisfactory when it can be shown that hallucination is possible—even necessary—on the basis of this being-disturbed or within the context of a disturbed existence" (van den Berg, 1982a, 103). Instead of hallucinations being seen as a sign of pathology, it is the presence of a disturbed state that predisposes us to look at the structure and function of imaginings. As we have seen, not all hallucinations are troublesome, nor is the general healthy population exempt from these outbursts of the imaginal.

Between self and other there is "no co-partnership, no discursive elucidation" (Straus, 1958, 166). Dialogue would be rare between such figures, as would the deepening of characterization. Contrary to claims that the hallucinated figures are so vivid that they rival perception, one finds that their characterization is shallow and superficial. The voice most often appears disembodied and motivations for the figure's actions are unarticulated, except from the external perspective—as in paranoid states when the habitual ego attributes motives to the figure.

> The schizophrenic hears voices, not persons. Occasionally, it is but one voice, but more often it is some, many or "they" voices emanating from an anonymous group: the Communists, the Masons, the Jews, or the Catholics. (Straus, 1966, 286)

The relation of the voices to other characters is not pursued. All focus is on the self.

> Understanding, shared or individual, demands some kind of indifference, the possibility of detaching oneself from the impact of impressions, of reflecting about oneself, of putting oneself into a general order in which places are interchangeable. (Straus, 1958, 166-167)

But in hallucinatory experience this interchangeability, this indifference and detachment are precisely those qualities that are absent.

In Sechehaye's *The Autobiography of a Schizophrenic Girl*, Reneé realizes when she begins to become well that not only have her hallucinations disappeared but the people around her are "no longer automatons, phantoms, revolving around, gesticulating without meaning," as were her hallucinated figures. "They were men and women with their own individual characteristics, their own individuality" (1951, 71). She says of her therapist:

> Mama too had changed in my eyes. Before she had appeared like an image, a statue that one likes to look at, though it remains artificial, unreal; but from this moment on she became alive, warm, animated, and I cherished her deeply. (71-72)

At the same time Reneé begins to feel as though she can influence things. She realizes for the first time that she can rearrange the furniture in her room: "What unknown joy, to have an influence on things; to do with them what I liked" (71). As her hallucinations recede, a passive ego role changes into a more active one, stereotypic figures into more animated and particularized ones.

In Hannah Green's account of schizophrenic experience, *I Never Promised You a Rose Garden*, a change in the nature of the relation between self and imaginal others signaled psychosis and the need for hospitalization. Initially Deborah had enjoyed the companionship of gods in an imaginal kingdom called Yr.

> Its gods were laughing, golden personages whom she would wander away to meet, like guardian spirits. But something changed, and Yr was transformed from a source of beauty and guardianship to one of fear and pain. (Green, 1964, 61)

Deborah then felt imprisoned in Yr. The Collect chanted curses at her, as she was "subject and slave to the Censor." "Once her guardian, the Censor now turned against her" (62). She did not challenge these characters as to the justness of their punishment and persecution of her, but suffered them passively during her period of greatest sickness. A crucial part of her therapy was her therapist's suggestion that she might take a more active role.

> The doctor rose to mark the session's end. "We have done very well this time, seeing where some of the ghosts of the past still clutch at you in the present." Deborah murmured, "I wonder what the price will be." The doctor touched her arm. "You set the price yourself. Tell all of Yr that it dare not compromise you in this search of ours." (113)

As Deborah began to fight the mercilessness of the Collect, becoming less passive, more distanced and reflective, the gods' characters changed again. Once again Deborah enjoyed their banter, wit, laughter and poetry. They became "amiable spirits" (268). For Deborah, successful treatment did not necessarily mean the disappearance of her gods, but an increased freedom to join in the world of other people, which entailed her being able to disobey her gods and stand firm against their relentless punishments. She differentiated herself from their rule.

The tyrannical and punitive nature of the voices in many hallucinations is also evidenced in *Perceval's Narrative: A Patient's Account of His Psychosis, 1830-1832* (Bateson, 1974). The period which led to Perceval's hospitalization was marked by voices commanding what he should do and think. When he would carry out their orders, the voices would criticize his attempts to obey, making him feel impotent and worthless. Perceval relates that during a year of his illness he scarcely uttered a syllable or performed an act that was not inspired by his "spirits." Perceval understood his cure as coinciding with a change in how he heard and understood the spirits, not with their disappearance. In short, he came to realize that "the spirit speaks poetically but the man understands it literally," that he was not supposed to do literally what his spirits had dictated but to hear them poetically. This shift from the literal to the metaphorical required a differentiation of self from the spirits so that command by the spirit and obedient action by the self was not a reflexive sequence. The self learned to stand apart from the spirits and hear them, rather than surrendering the ability to act and speak to the spirits. Straus remarks that it is no wonder that in many languages (Greek, Latin, Hebrew, French, German, Russian, English) "the words 'hearing' and 'obeying' are derived from the same root" (1966, 281). In English "to obey" stems from the Latin *obaudire* meaning to listen from below.

In an anthropological account of hallucinations, *The Spirit Possession of Alejandro Mamani* (Sanders, 1976), a Bolivian Indian commits suicide to escape the voice of a spirit. As his tribe was accustomed to hearing the voices of spirits, it was not the presence of the voice that drove him to desperation but the loss of his own freedom and autonomy with respect to the spirit. In short the voice would not stop speaking to him even when he tried to sleep. His activities and thoughts were constantly interrupted by the spirit's voice. He felt impotent, passive, and denuded of his agency. Ritual ceremonies did not give him distance from the voice, and so he turned to death as a means of silencing his tormentor.

It may at first appear contradictory to say that the person who is judged to be hallucinating may at the same time be both seeing the imaginal other egocentrically and feeling overwhelmed and threatened by the other's presence. Asking the person to hear the voice of the imaginal other might be seen as encouraging a toppling of the ego. But perhaps it is precisely the egocentric stance toward the voice that makes it seem so frightening (he or she is known only from one point of view), that increases its degree of insistence and intrusion into the conscious life of the "hallucinator." When a voice is finally listened to, and not just denied or struggled against, it frequently complains about how the imaginer never listens to it or takes it seriously.

Despite different metapsychologies (phenomenological, Jungian, psychoanalytic), a number of clinicians have turned to meet the voices of their patients, encouraging a more active and mutual relation between patient and voices. Lockhart, in "Mary's dog is an ear mother: Listening to the voices of psychosis," describes the treatment of a patient who had been hospitalized for head-shaking and auditory hallucinations. Lockhart reports that the patient felt "controlled" by the voice of his neighbor, Teresa, and complained of "being weary of being her puppet. He wanted nothing to do with her, resented this constant sexual battering and wanted to be rid of her" (1975, 149). Instead of focusing on the head-shaking behavior or reality testing, and instead of siding with the patient's desire to be rid of Teresa, Lockhart attempted to create an environment where the voice could be talked to and about. The clinical result was that the voice became less intrusive and the character of the imaginal figure changed from that of a controlling woman, preoccupied by sex, to a quasi-religious figure. The religious aspect, however, did not appear until the patient had satisfied in fantasy the sexual demands made by Teresa. A relation of control was transformed to one of greater mutuality. In Lockhart's words, "Once an individual begins to relate actively to the inner images, the controlling nature of these autonomous psychic processes is softened and often transformed" (1975, 152).

Medard Boss, in *Psychoanalysis and Daseinanalysis*, describes a series of attempts to treat an intelligent woman, suffering from visual and auditory hallucinations. At first Boss used Dubois' "persuasion" method, trying to help the woman "gain distance from the ugly visual and auditory phenomena by calling them mere hallucinations without any reality" (1963, 8): no success. Boss then treated them physiologically, as "expressions and results of a disturbed metabolism in the brain tissues" (8-9), showing the patient an EEG as proof, again with no success. The woman laughed at all his physiological and naturalistic explanations. Boss then conceded to his patient that her hallucinations "were not simply nothing," but insisted that they did not "correspond to an external reality, but represented only an internal, purely psychic reality, consisting of hidden emotions and tendencies of the patient herself" (10). He argued that these psychic realities were being projected onto external objects. But the patient did not accept this either, objecting to Boss' attempts to make mere fictions of the spying figures of her experience, to "dispose of them as mere hallucinations and projections of my own unconscious or some other psychic reality" (10). Much like Jung, Boss found himself turning to listen to the voices and to studying their materialization in the patient's drawings. The patient said her drawings "come out of nowhere, just suddenly appear, emerge from somewhere behind the drawing paper, and all of a sudden they are there, looking at me" (11). They are not experienced as internal voices but as beings who approach her from without, indeed who spy on her. The therapy began to move when Boss finally said to her,

> You are perfectly right. There is no sense in granting one reality priority over another. It would be quite futile for us to maintain that the fable before us is more real than your motorcycling spies merely because they elude my perception and are perceptible only to you. Why don't we let both of them stand as the phenomena they reveal themselves to be? Then there is only one thing worth our attention. That is to consider the full meaning-content of that which discloses itself to us. (13)

Boss begins to hear not just the woman's reality of being the victim of spies but to hear the reality of the spies—that is, that these spies occur because of two enemies, "mutually barred against each other and consequently antagonistic to one another, and where one party wants to annihilate the other or at least to conquer it and bring it under its own dominion" (13). From the spies' point of view the woman has been fighting them off as enemies. Boss, interpreting the war as the woman's rejection of her own erotic nature encourages her to stop fighting the spies: "Let the spies come and give them full power to do as they wish, and just see what happens" (14). Boss reports the woman now felt understood and placed her confidence in the treatment.

In each of these cases the voices initially sounded destructive, intrusive. But this was so not from the voices' point of view but from the ego's. As a mutual relation was fostered—in place of ridding, negating, defensive plays against the voice—it became possible to see what the imaginal figure wanted and how he or she saw the ego. In each case there was a granting of reality to the voice, and at the same time an attempt to hear it metaphorically, to satisfy it in fantasy. The voice's attempt to control is viewed finally in relation to how the ego is treating the figure, rather than as a contextless attack to be avoided by patient and therapist.

Of great importance is the fact that improvement was brought about not by arguing the priority of intersubjective reality over the preobjective reality of the imaginal (i.e., not by urgently attempting to ensure that the person could differentiate between percept and image). The work of doctor and patient was to understand the figure and to find a more reciprocal mode of relating.

CHAPTER TWELVE

The Fish-Lady and the Little Girl: A Case History Told From the Points of View of the Characters

Within every[one] there is an inconsolable child.
—Andre Schwarz-Bart

In a conversation between Tolstoy and Gorky, Gorky reports that [Tolstoy] rubbed his chest hard over the heart, raised his eyebrows, and then, remembering something, went on: "One autumn in Moscow in an alley near the Sukhariot Gate I once saw a drunken woman lying in the gutter. A stream of filthy water flowed from the yard of a house right under her neck and back. She lay in that cold liquid, muttering, shivering, wriggling her body in the wet, but she could not get up."

He shuddered, half closed his eyes, shook his head, and went on gently: "Let's sit down here... It's the most horrible and disgusting thing, a drunken woman. I wanted to help her get up, but I couldn't; I felt such a loathing; she was so slippery and slimy I felt that if I'd touched her, I could not have washed my hand clean for a month—horrible! And on the curb sat a bright, gray-eyed boy, the tears running down his cheeks: he was sobbing and repeating wearily and helplessly: 'Muum...mu-um-my...do get up.' She would move her arms, grunt, lift her head, and again—back went her neck into the filth."

He was silent, and then looking round, he repeated almost in a whisper: "Yes, yes, horrible! You've seen many drunken women? Many—my God! You, you must not write about that, you mustn't."

"Why?"

He looked straight into my eyes and smiling repeated: "Why?" Then thoughtfully and slowly he said: "I don't know. It just slipped out...it's a shame to write about filth. But yet why not write about it? Yes, it's necessary to write all about everything, everything." Tears came into his eyes. He wiped them away and smiling, he looked at his handkerchief, while the tears again ran down his wrinkles. "I am crying," he said. "I am an old man. It cuts me to the heart when I remember something horrible."

And very gently touching me with his elbow, he said, "You, too—you will have lived your life, and everything will remain exactly as it was, and then you, too, will cry worse than I, more 'streamingly,' as the peasant women say. And everything must be written about, everything; otherwise that bright little boy might be hurt, he might reproach us—it's untrue, it's not the whole truth,' he will say. He's strict for the truth." (1920, 80-82)

Tolstoy suddenly sees through the gray eyes of "that bright little boy" and reverses his stance. At first he had automatically sought Gorky's promise to ignore the drunken woman. Then through his streaming tears he becomes aware of the price of this ignorance—the little boy. With this insight, the boy begins to gain a voice which confronts Tolstoy. "It's untrue, it's not the whole truth." Tolstoy ends up wanting to write the truth as the boy lives it.

It is just such a shift—from Tolstoy's point of view to that of the character of the small boy—that distinguishes a psychotherapy which respects the autonomy and necessity of imaginal figures. In such a therapy one turns outside of the spontaneous and habitual ego responses to the characters in order to hear from them of their truths. The ego stance changes from ignoring to observing.

When thought is heard as dialogical the therapist's task becomes one of helping to make explicit the various voices it contains. As well as attending to "history" and the "literal" events of daily life, therapist and patient try to discover the multiplicity of imaginal histories and events which the characters make reference to and act from. As a result of these tasks case history can no longer be narrated by the therapist in an omniscient style, largely from an external point of view. Case history needs to reflect the psychic multiplicity uncovered in the therapy, allowing the characters to tell their stories from their own points of view.

Because in a case told from the characters' point of view the process of therapy recedes into the background, let me begin with some procedural details. In this kind of therapy the whole room is used as a place of enactment. There is freedom to move, to lie down on the floor, to enlist the therapist as a co-character, to scream or cry. This freedom is established to facilitate the unfolding of the characters.

The patient may speak about what has happened during the week, but there is often a move to who was involved imaginally—which characters—and how the event was seen from their different perspectives. In a way, one is asking "What is the dream of this event?" "What is the imaginal background?"

For instance if someone complains of depression, we need to know what the imaginal sense of the depression is and who, which character(s), suffer it. Is the scene of the depression a parched moonscape, an isolated bog of quicksand, or a bleak rooming house? Does one's depression express itself as an abandoned child, an aging man, a struggling single mother taking care of everyone? Even when the person identifies at first with the depression ("It is just me who is depressed"), he can often give hints to the images beneath: "I feel so old;" "I feel like I never want to leave my bed, like an invalid;" "I draw the curtains shut, so it will be like night inside." In some depressions, as in this case, the external picture may appear fine, "correct." He may have a job, primary relationship, friends, perhaps children. But within moments the individual may be painfully aware of not really feeling alive. Daily life may be experienced as a sequence of prescribed motions that "should"—are calculated to—give pleasure and fulfillment but do not.[37]

In the case presented here[38] of a woman in her late thirties, the depression was suffered by the character of a child.[39] When the

---

[37] Marion Milner (pseudonym Joanna Field) describes this kind of depression in *A Life of One's Own* (1981). See also Alice Miller's *The Drama of the Gifted Child* (1981).

[38] Gratitude is extended to "Laura" who allowed two years of her psychotherapy and imaginal dialogues to be audiotaped, transcribed, and shared here.

[39] For readers interested in pursuing the significance of the imaginal child, see Hillman (1973), Bachelard (1969), and Jung and Kerenyi (1949).

woman's thoughts were listened to closely the small child's voice could be heard.

Therapy usually commences with the presentation of the ego's point of view about what is wrong and how it might be "fixed up." Beginning active imagination and imaginal dialogues does not solve this dilemma, for one usually finds oneself taking the ego's point of view toward the characters. For instance with the imaginal child this often means that the child's demands are seen as "childish." One is willing to speak to the child now if there is a guarantee that by doing so the child will grow up and cease to be a nuisance. The child's feelings and wants are experienced as yet another burden to be navigated.

The woman, Laura, would initially be hopeful that the child would grow up. She would inquire about the child's age with eagerness, feeling a sense of improvement if the child said she was ten rather than eight and a sense of defeat if all at once the child turned baby or repeated the same scene at the same age over and over again.

The naturalistic development of a child growing up is not coincident with imaginal development. The first step in imaginal development is for the child's story to be heard more on its own terms, and less on the ego's. Several things can help promote this process. At times when the habitual ego's point of view and the child's are radically opposed, and one can tell it is not letting the child be heard without rushing in with objections and negations, one can have the child talk directly to the therapist. The therapist acts like a novelist might. She wants to know what the world is like to that character. She is interested in how the child sees the ego point of view and other relevant characters. Therapist and patient try to be like Conrad's narrators—persons in whom others feel compelled to confide. The characteristics of the narrator must, therefore, change as the confidant varies. In this case the child loved to talk in the session. When Laura talked the whole time, Little Laura was angry and would begin to ask for time for herself. A second helpful thing is to search out the personification(s) of the ego's point of view. Once it too can be treated as a character, whose perspective is important but only partial, the person's narrator can more freely arise. The narrator's position is like that of the therapist. He or she has less of an investment in any particular character over another and is more interested in the unfolding of the drama between the characters. The narrator is an observing presence who can reflect on and mediate between the other characters.

Let us try to begin our case from the characters' points of view.[40] Our story begins therefore with a young girl, "Little Laura," who felt chronically abandoned by my patient. Her father had died when she was a child. Her mother had not cherished her aliveness. Then she found herself with my patient, whom Little Laura reported most often ignored her, tried to lock her out of important life decisions (whom to marry, whether to have children, what to do professionally). At times she said she had felt so pushed out of the body and threatened with extinction that she had gotten my patient into physical accidents, partly as revenge for being so excluded. She thinks another character is trying to kill her by pushing her out of the body.

The woman the imaginal child spoke of, Laura, arrives at the first session of therapy depressed. She begins to cry. She has recently had her third child. During the pregnancy she began to feel more and more alone. She is now housebound again and separated from full involvement with her work. She struggles with her oldest child, with whom she often feels colder and tighter than she would like. "What is this marriage?[41] This family? This house?" she wonders—where she feels so alone, so far from fulfilling her ambitions? Too many responsibilities, too little time, too many things she wants to do—a story familiar to many women in their thirties, torn and bloodied by conflicts among the things they love. Who are the forces in this battle? Who first complains that life is not livable as it is currently arranged? Little Laura. Laura feels the sadness of this child and hopes that by paying her some attention she can be made to grow up and cease being so disruptive.

But when Little Laura is allowed to speak she makes it clear that her goal is not to grow up but to be allowed to live and exist. At first she feels almost dead and acts extremely passively.

> Something is draining off the juice and making me get smaller... Something is making me dizzy. I don't know

---

[40] The words of the characters, Laura, and the therapist are as originally spoken and recorded in the sessions.

[41] Hillman (1973) speaks of the necessary relation between the abandoned imaginal child and marriage: "Because every home established, every nest, niche or habit offers the abandoned child a sanctuary, marriage unavoidably evokes the child" (367).

where my weight is. I don't feel like myself anymore. Like someone's trying to sabotage me. And I feel stiff. I feel like someone is trying to kill me, to stop me from moving. Everything is atrophying, nothing is going to be any good anymore.

As we speak more to her she gives her own history, which borrows some events from Laura's life but puts different emphasis on them. For her the death of her father and her best friend are the most important events. The ego point of view thought that these events had been mourned enough, and would ask, "Will I always keep crying over this my whole life?"—fearful that she would become "stuck" on it. The little girl returns to her grief over this abandonment again and again. She feels that the father enjoyed and supported her liveliness, let her play spontaneously and was pleased by her inventiveness. When the little girl begins to feel more alive, she experiences at the same moment the deep sadness over the father's absence. If one sided with the ego's point of view, on this mourning—that it was possibly pathological—and did not give it space, one would be denying the child her liveliness. And so she cried and cried. The habitual ego point of view is mirrored in the character of the Manager or the Organizer. This organizing one finds crying about the dead father acceptable only if one cries and then never cries again. She feels "embarrassed over being attached to these dead people. It is indecent. "

The second part of the little girl's life that most preoccupied her was how she was never consulted about the major life decisions Laura had made: What job to take and how to do it, whom to marry, whether to have children, and if so how many. As our speaking with her seemed to bring her more to life, her depression took the form of anger. She felt the only way to survive was for Laura to leave her family behind. The child in a session speaks to me about Laura:

> *Little Laura*: I just don't think it is fair to let her win like this. It's just the same thing every time she gets to talk. And she talks about love, and intimacy and everything and then she wins, because those things are always allowed to win. Last time she went to a therapist she won. He said she should get closer to her husband and be more intimate with friends. She may say she doesn't want me to die, but she won't do anything. No one likes me anyway. There's no use talking. I don't want more time. I don't

> want to deal with it. I don't want to keep making all those compromises. I want to get out. This is the last straw. There is nothing left for me. I know I'm going to give in. I'll take what you give me, Laura, and try to make something with it.

Here Little Laura cries for a long time and then says,

> But it doesn't feel like I can do it. It doesn't feel like there is anything left. It feels like a fiction that I ever did anything. You can't keep doing nothing and expect that the thing will survive. If you don't do the work for years and years you're not that anymore. It's ridiculous.

When finally given a chance to speak she would rail against the conventions she assumed had blotted her out: marriage and motherhood.

> *Therapist*: So you feel betrayed by the compromises.
> *Little Laura*: Sure.
> *Therapist*: As though they were done just to appease you rather than having your interests in mind?
> *Little Laura*: Yes. They were done because I would insist on them sometimes. But when it comes to making a big decision about whether or not to have a baby, then I don't get to talk. She's [Laura] too strong. It's only if there are little decisions afterwards then I get to vote. So that when we were pregnant I could go take classes—well three weekends away doing a workshop. It really was a farce. I'm allowed to feel productive for a little tiny piece of time. It's not enough time, it's not enough to keep something going. It's just enough to keep the edge off. So I don't feel completely empty and dead, but I'm no fool. I get taken in by it and I feel a little better. I'll think I want to go away for a few days to work, but it is foolish. It is nothing real. I don't know what I want. What I'm saying is I want to quit. I don't want to have this family. It's just pissing me off that she can win by saying, "This feels good," or "I love somebody, "or you know, it's like that's the only thing that is important. It wins without explanation. I have to explain everything. If I want to do something I have to explain why it is important, it has to be part of a big plan. It's not enough for me to just want to live in another place or go someplace because I want to do it. I have to have a reason. It has to be part of a career plan, and she [Laura] doesn't have to have a reason. I don't

> know who it is we are explaining it to. But it is like there is somebody deciding who's right.
> *Therapist*: Like a judge.
> *Little Laura*: Yes, somebody who decides how the time is spent, whether it is more important to get the mold out of the refrigerator or get ready to do some work. I just don't think it is fair that she gets to win all the time.

For a long time Laura assumed that the child stood for her work, that the child wanted to leave the household to do intensive work. It was true that Little Laura was interested in some of the work, but she was not reducible to it. Equating the child with creative work was a way of justifying time spent with Little Laura to the Organizer. At times the child herself would use this rationalization. At other times, she was able to ask for attention without having to promise to produce things in return.

The third important thing to Little Laura was reliving her babyhood with her mother. The child as a baby does not want to move forward in space. She holds her breath and has a hard time talking. She says to her mother: "Are you going to stay? Will you lie down with me for a little while?"

> *Little Laura to Mother*: I want you to lie down with me, against my back. Put your arm around me…
> *Therapist to Little Laura*: What does your mommy say or do?
> *Little Laura to Therapist*: Oh, just that she wants to get on to the next thing.
> *Little Laura to Mother*: I want you to lie down next to me, and go to sleep…just close your eyes. I don't want you to look at me, I don't want you to think of me. Just lie down now and go to sleep. Don't think about anything. Nothing. You stay there…don't go… You stay there and don't go. I want it to be all dark. I want to lie there in the dark, and just be a shape. You wait. You can dream…but no thinking. OK? It's like we could be floating…like in a boat. You used to do it, you used to… Why not? But you did. I want you to be there right against my back. Like there is some kind of weight on my spine. I don't want you to be lying there and thinking about when you have to go.

It is tempting to understand this scene between a mother who does not want to just be with her child, who is driven to organize and do things, and a child who can hardly breathe or talk in her presence, as a metaphor for Laura's experienced relation to her actual mother. We could say that this essentially uninterested mother made the father's support all the more missed and longed for. That may well be so. However, it is also true that Laura has most often taken this role of abandoning busy mother to the imaginal child. She may promise to spend some time with the child, but this can be easily avoided by claiming to have lists of things to do or by merely not being present to the child during the appointed time. Abandonment by mother and the death of the father was not something solely in the past, but a daily situation for the child.

So far we have presented Little Laura in her abandonment, depression, despair and anger. But as the motif of the divine child in mythology and literature shows, these are accompanied by some sort of magic and wonder (see Jung and Kerényi, 1949).

Laura as Narrator did struggle to find time to spend with Little Laura. And as she became more successful at this—which meant being the go-between for Little Laura and the Organizer, the child and the woman who longed for the security of her family—the magic emerged. There began a process where Little Laura, who had been forced out of the body, began to take a part of it. When the child was given space in Laura's body, the body loosened, relaxed. At times, it felt as though the body and her energy were becoming huge, like a gigantic balloon, taking up the whole room. At other times the child was experienced as a region of the body, or as a round hole in the solar plexus that allowed direct entrance to the world. Little Laura was now open in spirit, loved to play, to imagine. She did not yell at Laura's children, but jostled and joked them into obedience. She ended up not always disliking the domestic scene and seeing it as her downfall, because as Laura allowed Little Laura to be present in her intimacy with her family, depression was lightened, and the time she spent with her family became more enjoyable, more pleasurable. Little Laura's demand that Laura leave her family had been very strong in the beginning. As Jung warned in his autobiography (1961, 187), it is extremely important not to literalize at first what a character asks for. Little Laura wanted life, and once this was more assured, she talked more lovingly of Laura's husband and children.

Unfortunately Little Laura was very vulnerable, and Laura's relation to her was tenuous to begin with. The Organizer was much more developed, and would squeeze the child out, taking over not only decision-making, but the body as well. Just as the actual mother had sent Little Laura back to the classroom after informing her of her father's death, so the Organizer left no time for feelings. It would take a while for the Narrator to realize that the body was tight and dead, Little Laura depressed and angry and the status quo strengthened. It was not enough to be on the side of Little Laura. In order to make room in her life for the spontaneity, creativity, and liveliness of the child, the Narrator needed to know inside and out the forces, the characters, who opposed the child. The characterization of each one was deepened as the others became more articulated.

At first we might see the Manager-Organizer as a dictatorial woman, immersed in a mania of doing, of endless details. She is tense and somewhat shallow, working like an automaton without a deep sense of meaningful priorities or heartfelt commitments. We might side too much with the little girl's anger against her. But just as we did not want to assume the absolute correctness of the ego's view of Little Laura, we do not want to accept as impartial the child's view of the Organizer. We want to move into the Organizer's autobiography and point of view.

One day Little Laura had been relentlessly demanding that Laura leave her home.

> *Little Laura to Laura*: You got to let me up. And I'm really going to give it to you and you're really going to have to do what I want. And that's going to mean that you really have to leave this time. You know there is no compromise. You are getting too old. This is too important.

The Organizer who wanted the home felt torn apart.

> *Organizer to Therapist*: I feel like everything will be torn into tiny little shreds, and that I won't be able to hold onto anything. It will all be in shambles. I just see this mess, this big mess. I feel like she is going to burst through me.
>
> There are little tiny pieces of paper and things are kind of floating, like there is no gravity. And things being shredded and fragmented. But as though the people were in pieces too.

THE FISH-LADY AND THE LITTLE GIRL

At one point when Little Laura was criticizing the Organizer, the latter said that she had to make her body stiff, because "otherwise I feel like I'm floating away and drowning." As the Organizer's vulnerability appeared, the Narrator could better protect her, and Little Laura, feeling more space, grew less bitter. Their warring would only recur when Laura had been out of touch with the child.

The Organizer also misses the father but is too afraid of these feelings to acknowledge them. She's afraid that her sadness and longing are intolerable. And so she sets about accomplishing things on lists, trying to keep up a pace that would not allow for feelings. As Laura spent more time with Little Laura, the Organizer appeared more reassured that the feelings would not overwhelm her, or destroy her home.

This awareness initiated a new phase in their relationship—one in which the Organizer did not stand in opposition to Little Laura and later to the Fish-Lady, but tried to aid them. And also, where the later characters of the Fish-Lady and the Narrator became more aware of the Organizer's values and fears. The other side of the Organizer's trying to accomplish things was her desire to be safe and protected. The Narrator says of her, "She is afraid of being hurt, afraid of doing things that will hurt her back, afraid that she won't get enough to eat. She will always make sure she eats something before she goes out of the house. She is meticulous about seeing that the children get enough to eat. If she is tired, she wants to go to bed."

Instead of experiencing the Manager or Organizer as a dictator, she begins to be seen as someone who tries her best but who needs help in order to make correct decisions. Her qualities of organization and planning begin to be admired.

> *Laura to Therapist*: I really need to keep up the dialogue with Little Laura. If I don't do it I feel like the Organizer always misinterprets things. She can't quite get it. It is always a little wrong in the direction of trying to make sense out of every single thing.
>
> It's almost like the Organizer doesn't have any sense of her own...just like a computer. So if I don't put in enough of the right information she gets it wrong and tries to make things orderly
>
> I'm afraid of her. I misinterpret too what she is doing. She'll set up an order of doing things and I'll say "Oh, OK we have to do this and that," instead of realizing that

she is just doing the best she can with what input there is. Every time I'm quiet about it and say "OK this is what we have to do" then it doesn't occur to her to ask me. And that's the problem, I wait to be asked. "Is this OK? How are you feeling? Are you still there?" And sometimes she just forgets to do that. She wants everything to be under control.

Little Laura also had initially felt sabotaged and drained, but was able through Laura's and the Narrator's attention to her to have periods of vitality where she gives freely back to the Narrator. She makes a joke, gives some advice and reassures. In one session the Narrator was anxiously inquiring how the child was: "Does she feel cheated or miserable?"

Little Laura to Narrator: I don't know why you expect me to be miserable. You seem to want me to feel bad. I feel fine. No, I don't feel miserable. You spent a long time talking to me this morning, and you've been talking to me every day. [Here there is a change. Little Laura for the first time responded to attention. She doesn't feel depressed or cheated despite the habitual ego's still thinking of her as weak.]

We're doing a lot of the work, I think. You're trying to find out where I am in your body, what helps me move around and go down deeper. That's all quite fun for me. I think you get all cramped up when you do the other work. [Here there is a beginning of reflection back to the Narrator.] You probably need some exercise or something to help you feel more released. As soon as you arrive in the morning you start working. You could take ten minutes and dance you know. Or fool around and you don't do it. Maybe I'm a little relieved not to have you pay so much attention to me. I feel like I'm getting stronger. This is a good relationship here. Here you've got a project to work on, and I can kind of work on my own and feel stronger and more solid without any danger that I'm going to miss anything. Later you'll spend more time with me.

Decision-making has gradually undergone a radical change. Whereas initially Little Laura was too weak to speak up, now the multiplicity is acknowledged by child, Narrator, and Manager. When a decision is to be made, one of them says "Hold it—a conference" and after each side has its say, some sort of compromise is worked out.

Little Laura is not just "in" an imagination, she has an imagination and loves to fantasize spontaneously. She did not want to be constrained to being in Laura's workroom or my therapy room. When asked where she would like to be or where she was, Little Laura had no difficulty describing the imaginal scene surrounding her.

> *Little Laura to Laura and Therapist*: I'm imagining Chris [Laura's son] and I are going sledding. It's a fairly big hill with lots of little hills. The snow is pretty deep. As we walk along he keeps falling down. He's singing. And then we pretend we are opera singers. [She sings aloud.] We sing back and forth to each other. Then we get up to the top of the hill. And then he gets scared of going down, and he says he doesn't think he can go down. But he is kind of enjoying being scared. Then I lay down on the sled and he gets on top of me. When we go down the hill it is very quiet, and late afternoon. There is a bump and he shrieks and yelps, and grabs on to me like he is going to fall off. When we get to the bottom there is an open field. He says, "Let's do it again, Let's do it again." I say, "Wait a minute I want to sit here for awhile." I have a battle with myself as to whether I want to really walk all the way back. Then it seems like the playing is over. He's a little tired. He keeps stopping to look at things as we walk home. Instead of walking back, we decided to walk through the woods.

As Little Laura gained in aliveness, assertiveness, and spontaneity, an interesting shift occurred. Laura went to the aquarium one day and realized that the "inner person who always wants to move is identified with a fish, where the tail moves as much as the rest of the body, the whole spine. That's the sort of motion she always wants to do. So sometimes now it feels like I've got a fish trapped inside of a cage, and the cage gets rigid sometimes and doesn't let the fish move at all." At first the Fish-Person alternated between being a Fish-Child and a Fish-Lady. Then there was a clear differentiation between the Fish-Lady and Little Laura. The Fish-Lady increased demands for movement and imagining. She was not concerned with the loss of her father any more—that was left to Little Laura. Little Laura wanted to move too, to jump and wriggle, but not in as sexual a way as the Fish-Lady did.

I purposely describe this development as a differentiation and not a split. From a psychoanalytic theoretical point of view this addition of another character would seem like a regression, since a goal is to integrate the voices into one. I, however, am approaching characters from a dramatic point of view. In drama, a single character can become more and more complex, but it cannot include in itself the full range of possible characters without losing the distinctiveness of each unique point of view. As the spontaneity and vitality of the child grew it was more aptly expressed as fishiness than as childishness. This did not mean that the child had grown up in some naturalistic fashion. Little Laura became more childlike and eventually became differentiated into two separate children.

As mentioned, the Fish-Lady demanded that Laura's life should include her even more.

> *Fish-Lady to Laura*: I don't understand. You figure all this stuff out and then you get into this trap where you can't feel good and you can't move around, and you think that every tiny concession you make to me is a big deal. I don't see why it is such a big deal. You feel as though what I want is unnatural or like there is something wrong about it, it's not something you'll let yourself go after. It seems to me like it ought to be like eating or sleeping. You treat it like it were a chocolate soda. Something real special that you can only do when there's a lot of time. I mean even if you don't have time to eat, you can have a snack, throw something in your mouth. I mean I guess that's what you've been doing the last couple of days.

The Fish-Lady voices her complaints against the Organizer to Laura and the Therapist:

> Like she—the Organizer—has the ability to decide what she wants and then she goes and does it. I don't have that ability quite. It's as though I don't have any legs. So I can only say what I need and then I have to get someone else to set me up to do it. And I feel like I ought to be growing legs but I don't know that I can do it any faster.

And the Organizer answers back:

> Well, I guess really that I don't like water, I don't like to get wet, or to be suspended, to be in a state where I don't have structure. I don't like not knowing what comes next. Like you got out on the porch to make a snow angel and

> you didn't know what to do next. That makes me uncomfortable. You're crawling around on the floor doing exercises and that makes you feel good, but I don't know what that leads to… I wish that you didn't need all that kind of thing. I wish that we could just go to work somewhere and go get a job, and have that separate from home. That way home and work would be separate. At night the job would be finished. This way I feel like you resent everything that I do, you resent every kind of job that I have to do. And I resent all of the demands you make. I feel like I have to give in to you or else you'll get really mad. I would like things to be more cut and dry. A list of things to do and then do them. And when I'm done with what I'm supposed to do then I could feel alright about it.
> *Laura to Therapist*: She's [the Organizer] saying she'd rather not have a body, but I think it is also not having any feelings. She holds her breath.

But the scenes of the first phase are still mainly there—namely, that there is a willingness on the Organizer's part to help out, if she knows what to do. Laura asks the Organizer:

> *Laura*: How do you feel if this stuff goes into my body and the Fish-Person gets bigger? And specifically if she gets a tail?
> *Organizer*: That would be great, because then I would know what to do.
> *Laura*: It's like the tail would be the thing that steers you.
> *Organizer*: You see I've been going around and planning things. You know. But I don't know where you want to go. I do it with the eyes. But if you just got down to your tail then you could steer it.
> *Laura to Therapist*: It was the first time she has been nice to this other one or even made a joke or anything. And then the next week I was feeling very high after some work. I said to the Fish-Person, "What would you eat under these circumstances?" The Fish-Person said: "Caviar and sushimi" [laughter], and that was her first joke.

Just as Little Laura had at first spoken only to Laura and had then practiced being present during our sessions, then with her family and then outside the home, so too the Fish-Lady began to want to go outside the confines of the work room and the therapy room. She says to me:

> *Fish-Lady*: I always like it if I get a chance to try something outside my room. Sometimes I try in the supermarket for a little bit.

But she fears that other people won't accept her:

> *Fish-Lady*: When I am with others, I can feel like I am drowning. Like I'm breathing in water like a fish and all of a sudden someone says, "My God, you're breathing water."

Still, she continues:

> *Fish-Lady*: I don't like the feeling of developing all this energy and then being all enclosed and alone. There is no way for it to travel. The image is that I need some kind of a corridor or a space or a direction. That I can see where it is going, so it is not just…so it can unfold into something else. I feel partly like I don't have any eyes yet. We've been working on my tail and back. But I can't see.
> *Therapist*: How could Laura help you with that?
> *Fish-Lady*: Maybe one thing I would like to do is go places and look at things I've never seen before. I get into a panic about what to do with the energy. I get to the edge of the room and there is nowhere to go. I need to see that there is something outside the boundary that I can go to. I get in a panic that there is nothing out there. So when the energy gets high I stop. I don't want to get sort of out and feel like I'm on a cliff [cries] and nowhere to go.
> *Therapist*: So Laura needs to bring in some things from outside or to take you out so there are some things to have dialogues with, to pull your energy in a certain direction.
> *Fish-Lady*: Yes. I don't like that feeling, where I feel like I'm alone [Fish-Lady cries].

It becomes clear to Laura how to bring forth the Fish-Lady:

> *Laura to Therapist*: I've been doing fine as long as what I am doing is to get the fishy side to be bigger, feel good, relax and it seems more and more that it is a lot of question of tension in the body. That once I relax certain muscles she just comes out. She's much more susceptible to that. I'll just start breathing or working on my spine and little by little I'll feel filled up. Often I'm only filled up to here and then I'll have to work on my neck, so she

comes also into my head. She is more alive and playful. I have spent a lot of time slowly trying to do that...

It feels like what I've been doing is working on the body so she can be more present, like taking the lid off the bottle so the genie can come out. And now it is like that feeling that the genie gets too big for the bottle, needs more room than the bottle.

Indeed the Fish-lady says, "I feel like my job is to get the body working again." She begins to make clear her priorities of being in a clear state, of "really feeling here."

> Fish-Lady: I don't feel like anything has happened until we've gotten into a certain state... Just saying, "Well how about if we work for an hour?" isn't enough. It could be that I just wander around the room or something.

The Fish-Lady pushes to clarify who becomes out of focus and sleepy during work times. It was often Little Laura who wanted her Daddy.

At times the clear "state" would occur outside the context of work and in the world.

> *Laura to Therapist*: I felt much more grounded in Washington than I usually feel. I felt like I was finding something out. It was just a feeling of being much more wherever I was all the time, like right in a place. Its that sort of feeling you have when details just sort of leap out at you, and you really just see where you are. It wasn't happening all of the time. There are times when I am in the mood and everything seems beautiful or like a painting. It wasn't like that. More of a feeling of weight, of feeling right there... I didn't feel like I had to run around all the time. I felt more than I ever do that I had some idea of what I wanted next all the time. Without having to wait for it... there weren't any in-between things going on. This time it was much more like breathing and eating. Then on the drive to Philadelphia, it was really an interesting feeling, sort of the same thing, but I was driving. It is almost like a texture, more than a feeling or a thought. I think it is like there is less distance between myself and the world, I have come out of myself more. The road felt closer. It felt like the car was lower down on the road. That I didn't have to go at a particular tempo, and if there was a jam at a toll booth, I didn't care, which is very unusual for me. I had the feeling that—I thought about what we had talked

about, about the quality of being abandoned. And at some point I said to myself on this drive, "I am my own father. I am going to take myself on this drive the way he would take me on this drive." And that's all. So I was doing for myself what I can do for my son.

What were some of the changes these imaginal dialogues encouraged? The presence of the imaginal child changed her relations with both her husband and her children, adding a certain playfulness and flexibility to daily events. Work, family and the wiggling movement of the fish did not seem necessarily antithetical anymore. Her work was re-grounded from a carrying out of what the Organizer thought she "should" do (a more superego, driven approach), to a waiting and nurturing of inspiration from Little Laura and the Fish Lady. Laura felt less torn apart by the conflicting points of view, though it was clear she needed to work to retain an awareness of the multiplicity of voices who shaped her inner life in order to maintain her energy and working relationships amongst the characters.

The depression which had opened the door to this drama gave way to emotional energy and bodily aliveness, as the voices were allowed to express themselves. Laura learned that more important than the results of her actions was to achieve a way of living daily life with the openness, vitality, and vibrancy so characteristic of the Fish-Lady. Before one becomes aware of the characters within thought and action, one often successively identifies with them, unconsciously becoming one and then another. For instance one spends the morning moving as the Organizer—frantically, breathlessly bringing to view other tasks to be done before the one at hand is completed. Then one lapses into the depression of Little Laura in the afternoon—that one who cannot yet feel her body, who is sensitive to abandonment. Once these identifications can be seen one can both begin to be aware of when the identifications are shifting and begin to interact with the particular characters rather than just being subject to them. One becomes aware that none of the voices can tell the whole truth, though each has an important story to relate. Dialogue with the characters can gradually supplant immersion in them. These shifts bring about the change from literal to psychological and metaphorical modes of understanding.

When one is identified with a character, let us say the abandoned child, reality ceases to be multifaceted. Reality becomes the child's reality, with all its instances and proofs of rejections, its moments of subjugation. When the narrating ego is taught to watch for identification and to dialogue with (or at least listen to) the characters' monologues, then "reality" can be seen from different points of view. From the perspective which sees thought as essentially dramatic therapy does not on all occasions aim at increasing identification and unification, but often at increasing differentiation and interaction. This experiencing of the self—as a collection of voices, organized through dialogue, observed by a narrating ego with a keen sense of metaphor—has its own stability, spontaneity, strength, flexibility, reliability, and continuity. It is a self which grows to tolerate conflict, ambiguity, and subtlety; a self which practices its empathy, humor, understanding and compassion on those within as well as those without.

Most often we see the imaginal from the ego's point of view. In the dialogues between Little Laura, the Fish-Lady and Laura, we caught occasional glimpses of how the characters saw the imaginal and how their points of view differed from that of the habitual ego.[42] For instance,

> *Little Laura to Therapist*: I'm the one that was there before all of these people started talking... I don't have all of those voices; it is the older one who has all of these. And I can help her if she just asks me what to do, because she can't tell sometimes. She gets a little afraid that there are too many. And even though she knows that it isn't crazy, it's like it sounds like something that could be crazy... She needs to remember that it just goes on in her head, and that really she has this very solid body. She lives in a place and she has these nice people whom she lives with and they love her. And those things, like those voices, are versions of things, but not one of them is everything.
>
> They are not everything and even if they fight with each other, she has to remember that the real part in the world is very ordinary and solid. She gets so that she feels she has to believe them, whichever one is talking and then she goes nuts, because the other one starts talking and she feels she has to do what that one wants. And then she thinks that they can't possibly live together if they want

---

[42] For additional commentary about how we treat voices—confining them to "inner space," failing to hear them, and inundating them with our psychologisms—see Hillman (1977).

both of those things. It's because she's pushing them to say the most extreme thing they can think of. It's not what they ordinarily ask. Once she comes out of there and plays a game with her daughter or talks to her husband or works, then she has fun, isn't forcing anything and it doesn't seem complicated. And I know that she wants to do that. I just think that sometimes she ought to ask me or something. I think it is easier when you let them all talk in their own voices. What drives you crazy is when you try to interpret everything. Interpret one of them to the other one, without really hearing exactly that one. Well, sometimes it's weird. Like the fat lady who talked last week was different from her saying "part of me wants to stay home, part of me wants to leave and work, part of me wants…" The fat lady didn't sound like part of her. It sounded like a completely different person. So that when she gets that way, it's not as crazy, it doesn't feel like she is demanding anything.

Therapist: If she can let herself be separate?

Little Laura: Even though it feels when you say it more strange, it really does make it less crazy.

Little Laura describes the imaginal as a group of voices each with its own version of things, no single one to be taken as truth in and of itself. Little Laura argues that the voices, although in Laura's head, are not just "part" of her. They need to speak in their own voices as separate people. From her perspective, craziness is interpreting the voices as part of oneself, denying them their autonomy. At the same time she does not belittle the day-world reality of body, family, and friends, but reminds Laura of them.

A year after this Laura had just emerged from a fight between the Fish-Lady and the Organizer. She said, "It's a relief to experience these things as separate. And…it seemed less confusing than when I would say I am arguing with myself, and it wasn't that differentiated. On the other hand, they seem stronger." So here differentiation does not serve a defensive function, diffusing affect, but results in clarifying the psychic scene and actually intensifying emotion.

When there is a lot of fighting and Little Laura feels like no one is paying her any attention, she says "I just begin to feel like I'm imaginary." For her the habitual ego, the Organizer, makes the real imaginary by ignoring it and devaluing it.

As the child is allowed to become real we find, as Jung did, that the child is both "all that is abandoned and exposed and at the same time divinely powerful; the insignificant, dubious beginning and the triumphant end. The 'eternal child' in mind is an indescribable experience, an incongruity, a handicap, and a divine prerogative" (1968c, § 300). This child, like others before her—Eros, Apollo, Proteus— found its Fish, in its own way and its own time. Development did not mean "growing up," but establishing conversations within which Little Laura, Fish-Lady, and the Organizer could be real and tell their own stories, their own truths.

As we have seen, the prevailing developmental theories assign imaginal dialogues to childhood. As Hillman points out, it is no wonder that therapy so often goes back to childhood,

> ...for that is where our society and we each have placed imagination. Therapy has to be concerned with the childish part of us (not for empirical developmental reasons) but in order to recreate and exercise the imagination. (1973, 168)

The drowning child caught in the undertow of a dream, an adult's piece of "childish" behavior that will not be extinguished, and a small child's voice that asks for Mommy in a moment of fantasy are often our entrances into imaginal dialogues. The child within us is accustomed to speaking out to animals and puppets, to those who have died and those who are absent, to those invisible guests who grace our table of thought. May we listen for their voices!

Psychotherapy may continue to help reflect and perpetuate the sociocultural bias against imaginal dialogues by continuing to mislabel experiences of the imaginal, assigning many of them a pathological status, discouraging the reporting (and perhaps the conscious experiencing) of thoughts' many conversations. It can continue to see psychic multiplicity solely as the product of schizoid operations, "hearing voices" as nothing but an aberrant mode of mind. But we will continue to dream. We will continue to fantasize. We will continue to speak to ourselves and others in the privacy of our thought. We will continue to take on others' voices and intonations, and we will continue at times to act and speak in ways that surprise us—as though for the moment we have given over our place to another.

We will continue to dream, and the dream will show us that beneath our cultural organization of self and conceptions about thinking, thought spreads itself out before us as imaginal scenes filled with characters and situations which are not always mere representations of what has already been experienced.

Psychotherapy need not always go from the dream's characters to thought and its associations, but can also move from thought to its scenes and characters—so thinly disguised are they, so ready to speak. The dramatic form employed by some psychotherapies is not a form or a technique applied to thought and feeling, nor is it an appropriate form simply because it reflects our dialogical relation to others in the world. Drama arises from and expresses the structure of thought itself, with its multiplicity of figures and viewpoints, and its lifelong conversations.

EPILOGUE

The very din of imaginal voices in adulthood—as they sound in thought and memory, in poetry, drama, novels and movies, in speech, dreams, fantasy and prayer—has led us to question the efficacy of contemporary developmental theories for fully understanding imaginal dialogues. These theories would lead us to believe that the imaginal dialogues of children's early speech and play are largely subsumed by the dialogues of social discourse and the monologues of abstract thought. Where they persist into adulthood they are most often seen either as pathological or as a means of rehearsing and rehashing social interaction (i.e., in service to shared reality). While not denying that imaginal dialogues play roles in the child's development of self-regulation of behavior, abstract thought, and language skills, and that imaginal dialogues supplement a deficient "reality" which often falls short of wish, we have questioned whether these are their only functions.

It has been suggested that these dialogues not only reflect, distort or prepare for the common reality of social interaction, but that they are creative of imaginal worlds and imaginal relations as well. These can be valued not just as subordinate to social reality, but as a reality as intrinsic to human existence as the literally social. The value and power of this imaginal reality has been severely circumscribed, and at times castrated, by the presuppositions of the modern scientific outlook which our developmental psychology shares. Developmental psychology has lent its weight to prevailing social conventions that dictate the permissible and impermissible forms of speaking with and through imaginal figures. Thus to reawaken a sense of value for imaginal dialogues we have of necessity gone outside the bounds of this scientific outlook to literature, mythology, and religion—regions where these dialogues have not had a peripheral significance, but a central one.

Here we do not find that imaginal dialogues disappear in time, as they are converted or subsumed into higher forms of thought. The characters do not become less multiple, less articulated, less autonomous, or more silent. One line of development suggested by literature, mythology, and religion is that imaginal figures become more released from the dominion of the self (i.e., more autonomous), more articulated, and more differentiated through their multiplicity. Interactions with these imaginal figures develop from monologue to dialogue—to relations which are reciprocal, where the integrity of each party is maintained. Our unearthing of this other developmental fate should not be taken as a rigid prescribing of *teloi*, but as an alternative way of approaching imaginal dialogues which liberates them, particularly those of adulthood, from a place of censure. When the spontaneous dialogues of thought are approached from this point of view they flower into drama, poetry, or prayer. Far from revealing themselves as a primitive form of thought, these dialogues reveal the complexity of thought as it struggles between different perspectives, refusing to be simplified and narrowed to a single standpoint.

Although our focus has been unremittingly on "imaginal dialogues," the subtext of this discussion has been an examination of the effect of developmental and scientific theory on our conceptions of the imaginal in general. To those who value the imaginal the word "development" has come to have the face of an enemy, of one who derogates, belittles, explains away, calls names. From a position of respect, both for what the concept of development can mean and for the experience of the imaginal, I have tried to show where they may begin to meet, such that a developmental approach to the imaginal need not eliminate its very subject.

AFTERWORD

On "Holding Holy Converse" with the Stranger: The Development of the Capacity for Dialogue

Buber teaches us that in the Hasidic apprehension of reality "a divine spark lives in every thing and being, but each such spark is enclosed by an isolating shell. Only man can liberate it and re-join it with the Origin: by holding holy converse with the thing and using it in a holy manner" (1970, 5-6). As I read back over *Invisible Guests*, now fourteen years since its initial publication, I can hear my own attempts to describe a manner of relating to the other that I could call "holy." For in the end, the developmental path I prescribed aims at the allowing of the other to freely arise, to allow the other to exist autonomously from myself, to patiently wait for relation to occur in this open horizon, to move toward difference not with denial or rejection but with tolerance, curiosity, and a clear sense that it is in the encounter with otherness and multiplicity that deeper meanings can emerge. It is through this manner of dialogue with the stranger that liberation and re-joining can occur.

I came to this sensibility through a sustained gaze on the unfolding of imaginal relations, particularly what I would call dialogical ones. Now, fourteen years later, I want to underscore what is mainly implicit in this text. Namely, that this manner of holy converse describes equally as well our relations with others, as it does our relations with ourselves, imaginal others, the beings of nature and earth, and that which we take to be divine. Relationships with imaginal others that are dialogical—in the ways defined here—are, in truth, a sub-text of "holy converse" more generally.

When we emphasize this frame there are a number of developmental theorists whose work bespeaks the interpenetration of these domains in terms of the development of dialogical capacity: for example, the peer therapy of Robert Selman; the work with adolescent girls of Carol Gilligan and her colleagues; the work with women's ways of knowing of Mary Belenky and her colleagues; the large group dialogue work of David Bohm and Patrick de Mare; and, finally, the liberational pedagogy of Paulo Freire. I will turn to these as exemplars to help us see some of the developmental threads that crisscross between dialogical domains, and to establish signposts beyond this text for those who wish to pursue the cultivation of dialogue.

The Capacity to Play and the Capacity to be a Friend: Differentiating and Coordinating the Perspectives of Self and Other

Klein and Winnicott, among others, noted that some disturbed children have an incapacity to play, which psychotherapy must address. In Winnicott's words: "...where playing is not possible then the work done by the therapist is directed towards bringing the patient from a state of not being able to play to a state of being able to play" (1971, 138). Selman and Schultz, working with the interpersonal relations of emotionally disturbed children, have noted that interactive fantasy play is markedly absent in the history of children whose interpersonal understanding is at primitive levels. These children do not understand that self and other can interpret the same event differently; i.e., the other is not understood to have an interiority different from my own. They are unable to differentiate between an unintentional act of another and an intentional one (the action is equated with the intent). Neither do they differentiate physical from psychological characteristics of the person (i.e., if the person is deemed pretty then she is a good person). In short, they are unable to "differentiate and integrate the self's and the other's points of view through an understanding of the relation between the thoughts, feelings, and wishes of each person" (1990, 6).

This capacity to differentiate and integrate the self's and the other's points of view is at the core of dialogical capacity. As Selman and

Schultz point out, a deficit in this ability shows both in problematic interpersonal relating and in an absence of the dialogues of pretend play. However, he also describes how the seeds for interpersonal dialogue can be planted in the dialogues of play. In his pair therapy work with children who are isolated by their own patterns of withdrawal or aggression, he pairs a submissive, withdrawn child (self-transforming style) with a child who is overcontrolling, sometimes downright bullying (other-transforming style). Initially they each cling to his or her own style, making impossible a deepening of relationship. Selman and Schultz share an image from a session with two such boys where one traps the other in the up position on the seesaw. There is no movement! In pretend play these two boys initially replicate their roles on the seesaw:

> Andy initiated a fantasy in which he was the television/comic book character "The Hulk," a large, powerful, fearsome mutant who is good inside, but who cannot control his feelings to let the good direct him. Paul then took a part as "Mini-Man," a being of his own creation who is smaller than anything else in the world and can hide in flowers... The play was a fantasy in which one boy had the power to control the thoughts and will of the other by virtue of a psychological "force-field. (169-170).

With these roles personified, however, each boy is as though seduced into wanting to embody each of the available roles. Paul experiments with putting up his force-field and then with "zapping" his partner, just as Andy relaxes his grip on power and enjoys the submissive position of "Mini-Man."

> Theoretically speaking we believe that this switching of roles in play is a key therapeutic process, in effect a way to share experience. Andy was able to relax his defenses and express the message that part of him was happy to be or even needed to be controlled, taken care of, told what to do. He could abandon for the moment the tenderly held goals for which he generally fought so fiercely... And Paul, often too frightened to take the initiative in actual interactions, was able to take steps toward assuming the control that he felt was too risky in real life, despite its practical and emotional attractions... When it is just play, children can dress rehearse for changing roles on the stage of real-life interaction. (171)

Here we see the interrelation between the dialogues of play and those of social discourse. Now, rather than "inner speech" being the internalization of actual social discourse, as in Vygotsky's theory, we see the dialogues of play as the seed that travels up into the soil of friendship and collaboration. Indeed, in Selman's third year of work with these boys, we see them able to withstand the storm of each other's emotions, to venture into different roles with one another, and to begin to share around the deepest area of each boy's concern.

Sustaining One's Voice Amongst Others

For authentic dialogue to occur it is not enough for one to be able to differentiate one's perspective from the other and to allow the other a voice. One must also be able to maintain one's own voice amidst the fray of relationship. In Chapter Eleven this was addressed in the domain of imaginal dialogues in the treatment of hallucinatory experience where, too often, the most disturbing aspect of hallucinatory experience is not a confusion of perception with image but a disavowal of the ego's point of view as it is swamped by the voice(s) of the other. The other's command becomes the self's action.

Carol Gilligan and her colleagues, in turning their attention to normative development in preadolescent and adolescent American girls, unfortunately found that not all the changes they witnessed in girls were ideal. One the one hand, they found that:

> As these girls grow older they become less dependent on external authorities, less egocentric or locked in their own experience or point of view, more differentiated from others in the sense of being able to distinguish their feelings and thoughts from those of other people, more autonomous in the sense of being able to rely on or take responsibility for themselves, more appreciative of the complex interplay of voices and perspectives in any relationship, more aware of the diversity of human experience and the differences between societal and cultural groups.

On the other hand they found:

> that this developmental progress goes hand in hand with evidence of a loss of voice, a struggle to authorize or take seriously their own experience—to listen to their own voices in conversation and respond to their feelings and

> thoughts—increased confusion, sometimes defensiveness, as well as evidence for the replacement of real with inauthentic or idealized relationships. If we consider responding to oneself, knowing one's feelings and thoughts, clarity, courage, openness, and free-flowing connections with others and the world as signs of psychological health, as we do, then these girls are in fact not developing, but are showing evidence of loss and struggle and signs of an impasse in their ability to act in the face of conflict. (Brown and Gilligan, 1992, 6)

In order to maintain the semblance of relationship these girls were struggling with "a series of disconnections that seem at once adaptive and psychologically wounding, between psyche and body, voice and desire, thoughts and feelings, self and relationship" (7). Too often girls were found stepping away from articulating their thoughts and feelings if these would bring them into conflict with others. What was initially conscious public disavowal of thoughts and feelings, over time became unconscious disclaiming. Girls then expressed that they felt confused about what they thought and felt, that they were unsure. Over time, many took themselves out of authentic relationship—with others and themselves. They became unable to identify relational violations, and thus were more susceptible to abuse. Brown and Gilligan began to wonder if they were "witnessing the beginning of psychological splits and relational struggles well documented in the psychology of women" (106).

To encourage girls' resistance and resilience Gilligan and her colleagues realized that it was not enough to help girls put into words for others their thoughts and feelings. For many, the fear of how their thoughts and feelings would be received had already metamorphosed into the girls' not listening to themselves. And so the women working with these girls tried to find ways to help the inner ear not go deaf and to revive a capacity to listen to one's selves, while at the same time building a group where the girls could experience that others can survive their voice(s): that authentic dialogue is possible, not just false or idealized relations.

Akin to Selman's move toward play, Gilligan's team moved toward supporting the girls' diary and journal writing, their dramatic and poetic writing, and their literally claiming their voices in their work.

Dialogue—in the ideal sense—necessitates both the capacity to deeply receive the other and the capacity to receive oneself; to allow the other a voice and to allow the self voice.

Being Silenced vs. Opportunities for Dialogue: Voice, Mind, Relationship, and Social Action

Belenky, Clinchy, Goldberger, and Tarule (1986), in *Women's Ways of Knowing: The Development of Self, Voice, and Mind*, vividly describe the interpenetration of dialogical domains addressed here as they study different ways of women's knowing. In one group of women they studied women's silence in adulthood was linked to family experiences of neglect and abuse. These women were passive, subdued, and subordinate in adulthood. "The ever-present fear of volcanic eruptions and catastrophic events leaves children speechless and numbed, unwilling to develop their capacities for hearing and knowing" (1986, 159). These women experienced themselves as mindless and voiceless. Their childhoods were not only lived in isolation from their family members and others outside the family, but most often were lived without play. The intersection of an absence of dialogue with an absence of play turned out to be particularly damaging for these children as they grew to womanhood.

> In the ordinary course of development, the use of play metaphors gives way to language—a consensually validated symbol system—allowing for more precise communication of meanings between persons. Outer speech becomes increasingly internalized as it is transformed into inner speech. Impulsive behavior gives way to behavior that is guided by the actor's own symbolic representations of hopes, plans, and meanings. Without playing, conversing, listening to others, and drawing out their own voice, people fail to develop a sense that they can talk and think things through. (1986, 33).

Moreover, the world becomes a place of simple dichotomies—good/bad, big/little, win/lose—obscuring all subtlety and texture.

Without play or dialogue the child is constrained within a narrow band of reality. Both play and dialogue allow the child to visit the perspectives of others, as well as to dream of that which has not yet come into reality. "What is" and "who one is" become radically widened as one de-centers from the ego's perspective and the given. Through the metaphorizing of play one leaps past the given confines of "self" and "reality." The dialogues of play and the dialogues of social interaction are both creative of the self and the liberating the self. Through each empathic leap, through each re-embodiment of ourselves in play, we pass beyond our usual borders and exceed what has been. What "is" is surpassed by what might be, and "who" I am is replaced by my transit beyond myself—either through projection of the self or through the reception of the other. Working an issue through play—expressing it, addressing it from several perspectives, taking the role of the others in play—is translated into the dialogues of thought and those of our everyday interactions. It should come as no surprise that the complexity and subtlety of a child's play, her flexibility in moving between the *dramatis personae*, can be seen in her participation in dialogue and in her capacities for reflection.

Childhoods that do not give opportunity for pretend play, where families discourage dialogue and where schools limit the classroom experience to verbal exchanges that are unilateral and teacher initiated, make it highly unlikely that children will learn the "give and take of dialogue" (Belenky *et al.*, 1986, 34), giving them access to what lies beyond a narrow self which has been schooled for silence. For such children, and the adults that are generated from them, words have force only when uttered violently. Thus they "tend to be action-oriented, with little insight into their own behaviors or motivations. Since they do not expect to be heard they expect no response, the volume of their voices is more important than the content. They lack verbal negotiating skills and do not expect conflicts to be resolved through non-violent means" (1986, 160). Those who do not escape silence pass the legacy of their early homes onto their children:

> Mothers who have so little sense of their own minds and voices are unable to imagine such capacities in their children. Not being fully aware of the power of words for communicating meaning, they expect their children to know what is on their minds without the benefit of words. These parents do not tell their children what they mean by "good"—much less why. Nor do they ask their children to explain themselves...
>
> We observed these mothers "backhanding" their children whenever the child asked questions, even when the

questions stemmed from genuine curiosity and desire for knowledge. It was as if the questions themselves were another example of the child's "talking back" and "disrespect." Such a mother finds the curious, thinking child's questions stressful, since she does not yet see herself as an authority who has anything to say or teach. (1986, 163-164)

These women were not aware of any experience within themselves of dialogue with a self or of having an inner voice; nor did their words express a familiarity with introspection or a sense of their own consciousness.

Those women in Belenky's study who were able to emerge from silence into adulthood had the benefit of a school which encouraged the cultivation of mind and an interaction with the arts, had been able to forge significant relationships outside the home despite the prohibition not to do so, or had "created such relationships for themselves through the sheer power of their imaginations, by endowing their pets and imaginary playmates with those attributes that nourish the human potential" (1986, 163).

In the other ways of knowing that Belenky *et al* describe—received knowing, subjective knowing, procedural knowing, and constructed knowing—intrapsychic and interpersonal dialogue are intimately related to each other, together forming a sense of flatness or complexity of reality. For instance in received knowing women experience others as the authority, silencing their own voices to be better able to imbibe the wisdom of others. It is not surprising that they seek to eliminate ambiguity from their worlds and can be described themselves as literal-minded. On the other hand, subjective knowers conceive of all truth arising internally, stilling their public voice, and often turning a "deaf ear to other voices." Often distrusting words, they cover disagreement with conformity and live in the isolation of their own thoughts and inner voices.

In what is clearly their preferred developmental *telos*, Belenky and her colleagues describe those who experience constructed knowing. In this way of knowing, knowledge is contextual. There are multiple viewpoints to be had, but not all are equally adequate to revealing what one is trying to understand. These knowers are familiar with listening to the inner voice or voices. Yet they know that even an inner voice may be wrong at times, for it is but one part of a whole.

They are also adept at patient listening to the voices of others. They have a high tolerance for internal contradiction and ambiguity.

Just as the child breaks the confines of the given through the dialogue of play, so too may the adult who can move between perspectives and systems of knowing. Liberated from subservience to external authority, to any one system of thought, and from slavish devotion to their internal voices, these knowers have the dialogical tools to break the oppressive aspects of "reality." Their nurture, care, and engagement with their own voices, the voices of others, and ideas broaden out to their nurture and care of aspects of the world.

From Cultures of Silence to Libertory Dialogue: The Work of Paulo Freire

This connection between coming to see the context one is in, gaining voice in relation to this context, and being able to creatively engage in efforts to effect culture is beautifully articulated in the work of Paulo Freire. Here silence and lack of dialogical capacity is understood to arise through oppression, which purposely creates voicelessness and obscures context in order to maintain power. Freire, the founder of the literacy movement in Brazil and radical pedagogist, argues that for the disenfranchised, learning to read should involve a process of becoming able to decode the cultural and socioeconomic circumstances that shape your life and your thinking. Once able to decode these conditions one is then able to participate in the shaping of those circumstances. He called the first step in this empowering process "conscientization," a group process which allows one to actively engage with the structures one has previously identified with and been blind to.

In Freire's model an "animator" helps group participants to question their day to day experience, their concerns and suffering, exploring the relation between daily life and the cultural dictates that suffuse it. Here words, much like play for the child, begin to open up the realm of the possible, liberating "reality" from the bonds of the given. Efforts at change are directed not foremost to the individual level, but to wider cultural change that will, in the end, effect the participants. This change becomes possible through the second step of Freire's method, "annunciation." Once a group knows how to decode the dominant paradigm and its effects—through having spoken together—then they can begin to conceive of social arrangements which are more just through the process of dialogue.

Why is this process necessary? Freire says that the dominant class attempts "by means of the power of its ideology, to make everyone believe that its ideas are the ideas of the nation" (Freire and Faundez, 1989, 74). A dominant paradigm operates by way of the monologue, not dialogue. It requires voicelessness on the part of the other to sustain itself. "The power of an ideology to rule," says Freire, "lies basically in the fact that it is embedded in the activities of the everyday life" (*Ibid.*, 26-27).

It is through dialogue that one breaks out of the "bureaucratization" of mind, where there can be a rupture from previously established patterns. "In fact, there is no creativity without *ruptura*, without a break from the old, without conflict in which you have to make a decision" (Freire, in Horton and Freire, 1990, 38). For Freire true education is not the accumulation of information placed in the student by the teacher. True education must encourage this rupture through dialogue. Teacher and student must each be able to effect, to communicate with, and to challenge each other, rather than perpetuate domination through monological teaching methods that further disempower.

Freire connects dialogue with love:

> Dialogue cannot exist, however, in the absence of profound love for the world and for [women and] men. The naming of the world, which is an act of creation and re-creation, is not possible if it is not infused with love. Love is at the same time the foundation of dialogue and dialogue itself. It is thus necessarily the task of responsible subjects and cannot exist in a relation of domination. Domination reveals the pathology of love: sadism in the dominator and masochism in the dominated. Because love is an act of courage, not of fear, love is commitment to [others]. No matter where the oppressed are found, the act of love is commitment to their cause—the cause of liberation. And this commitment, because it is loving, is dialogical... (Freire, 1970, 77-78)

AFTERWORD

Dialogue Across Difference: Bohm's Large Group Dialogue

In Freire and Faundez's work the concept of culture is not linked to ideas of unity but to diversity and tolerance. This shift toward the acknowledgment of diversity invites voices to speak which have been marginalized by the dominant culture and its paradigms. This movement from center to margin requires a process of dialogue that assumes difference and seeks to articulate it. Truth is not located in a particular perspective, it "is to be found in the 'becoming' of dialogue" (Faundez, in Freire and Faundez, 1989, 32).

David Bohm, physicist and colleague of Krishnamurti, describes a kind of large group dialogue where it is through the difference that is present that one can begin to hear one's own assumptions. Bohm asks that once we hear these assumptions we try to suspend them rather than using our characteristic defensive moves of overpowering the other voices, defending our assumptions as the truth. This acknowledgment and suspension of assumptions is done in the service of beginning to see what it is one means. When we defend an assumption, says Bohm, we are at the same time "pushing out whatever is new... There is a great deal of violence in the opinions we are defending" (1990, 15). Through coming to see our own and others' assumptions we arrive at a place where we can begin to think together, seeing more of the totality that comprises our situation. Sampson is careful to remind us that allowing others to speak is not enough if they cannot "be heard in their own way, on their own terms," rather than be constrained to "use the voice of those who have constructed them" (1993, 1220-1223).

Here one is required to take a third-person point of view towards oneself, reflecting on how one's actions, attitudes, and assumptions arise from particular ideologies. And further, how the ideologies we are identified with have effected the other, the stranger.

Like imaginal dialogues, such dialogue in a large group requires the suspension of usual egoic modes of operation: judging, condemning, deeming oneself superior (or inferior). These interfere with listening deeply, with the radical entertaining of the other, which at the same moment can awaken us to where we each stand.

Coda

In the end, the direction of this book is not inward...only. It cannot be, because imaginal dialogues do not exist separate from the other domains of our lives. The hierarchies of our culture, schools, family—and thus of mind—do not deeply invite dialogue. Neither does the voicelessness directly resulting from such hierarchies of power. Here I am trying to underscore the interpenetration of dialogues with imaginal others, with dialogues with oneself, one's neighbors, within one's community, between communities, and with the earth and its creatures. The effort to section off the imaginal from this larger fabric is at best defensive and at worst wasteful of the energies needed to work at much-needed reconciliations. Depth psychology—if it is not to become a Euro-American relic from the nineteenth and twentieth centuries—must use its energy to penetrate the depths of difference. Dialogue is the method for this hosting, penetration, and holding of difference.

For the sake of dialogue—of love—this book points us toward the creation of childcare contexts where the dramatic fray of play can be delighted in, to elementary schools where the leap between self and others in a small group can be practiced, to spiritual education and practice where the voices within silence can be discerned and addressed. It points us toward high schools and colleges where previously marginalized voices can be admitted to the mosaic, changing the underlying structure of education from the conveyance of dominant paradigms to one of dialogue across difference. It turns us toward the processes of non-violent communication and reconciliation that are needed to nurture the neighborhoods and communities—and ultimately nations—in which we are homed. And finally, it attempts to turn us toward the dialogue beyond words required between nature and humans if our actions are to finally preserve the earth.

REFERENCES

Abrams, M. L. (1953). *The Mirror and the Lamp: Romantic Theory and the Critical Tradition*. New York: Norton.

Anthony, E. J., (1975). "Naturalistic Studies of Disturbed Families." Ed. E. J. Anthony. *Explorations in Child Psychiatry*. New York: Plenum Press.

Arendt, H. (1971). *The Life of the Mind*. New York: Harcourt Brace Jovanovich.

Arrowsmith, N., and Morse, G. (1977). *A Field Guide to the Little People*. New York: Pocket Books.

Austin, J. L. (1962). *Sense and Sensibilia*. Oxford: Oxford UP.

Avens, R. (1980). *Imagination is Reality: Western Nirvana in Jung, Hillman, Barfield, and Cassirer*. Dallas: Spring Publications.

Bachelard, G. (1969). *The Poetics of Reverie*. Boston: Beacon Press.

Ball, B. (1883). *Leçons sur les Maladies Mentales*. Paris: Asselin.

Barten, S. (1983). "The Aesthetic Mode of Consciousness." Eds. S. Wapner and B. Kaplan. *Toward a Holistic Developmental Psychology*. Hillsdale, New Jersey: Lawrence Erlbaum Associates.

Bateson, G., ed. (1974). *Perceval's Narrative: A Patient's Account of his Psychosis, 1830-1832*. New York: William Morrow.

Belenky, M., B. Clinchy, N. Goldberger, and J. Tarule (1986). *Women's Ways of Knowing*. New York: Basic Books.

Beres, D. (1965). "Symbol and Object." *Bulletin of the Menninger Clinic*, 29, 3-23.

Beres, D., and Joseph, E. (1970). "The Concept of Mental Representation in Psychoanalysis." *International Journal of Psycho-Analysis*, 51, 1-9.

Bion, W. R. (1962). *Learning from Experience*. New York: Basic Books.

⎯⎯⎯⎯⎯⎯ (1963). *Elements of Psycho-analysis*. New York: Basic Books.

Blatt, S. J., and Wild, C. M. (1967). *Schizophrenia: A Developmental Analysis*. New York: Academic Press.

Bleuler, E. (1951). "Autistic Thinking." Ed. D. Rapaport. *The Organization and Pathology of Thought*. New York: Columbia UP.

Bohm, D. (1990). "On Dialogue." Ojai, Calif.: David Bohm Seminars.

Boleslavsky, R. (1933). *Acting: The First Six Lessons*. New York: Theatre Arts.

Boss, M. (1963). *Psychoanalysis and Daseinanalysis*. New York: Basic Books.

Bowen, E. (1975). *Pictures and Conversations*. New York: Knopf.

Bradley, A. C. (1920). *Oxford Lectures on Poetry*. London: Macmillan.

Brierre de Boismont, A. (1859). *On Hallucinations*. Trans. R. T. Hulme. London: Henry Renshaw.

Brown, L. and Gilligan, C. (1992). *Meeting at the Crossroads*. New York: Ballantine Books.

Buber, M. (1915). *Daniel*. Leipzig: Insel-Verlag.

_____ (1958). *I and Thou*. New York: Scribner's.

_____ (1970). *The Way of Man*. New York: Citadel Press.

Bundy, M. W. (1927). *The Theory of Imagination in Classical and Medieval Thought*. Urbana: University of Illinois, Studies in Language and Literature.

Burke, K. (1945). *A Grammar of Motives*. Berkeley: University of California Press.

Carver, R. (1981, February 15). "A Storyteller's Shoptalk." *The New York Times Book Review*.

Cary, J. (1958). *Art and Reality*. Cambridge: Cambridge UP.

Casals, P. (1967). *Casals, a Living Portrait*. Columbia Records.

Casey, E. S. (1971-1972). "Freud's Theory of Reality: A Critical Account." *Review of Metaphysics*, 25, 659-690.

_____ (1976a). "Comparative Phenomenology of Mental Activity: Memory, Hallucination, and Fantasy Contrasted with Imagination." *Research in Phenomenology*, VI, 1-25.

_____ (1976b). *Imagining: A Phenomenological Study*. Bloomington: Indiana UP.

Cassirer, E. (1955). *The Philosophy of Symbolic Forms, Vol. II: Mythical Thought*. New Haven: Yale UP.

Chambliss, J. J. (1974). *Imagination and Reason in Plato, Aristotle, Vico, Rousseau and Keats*. The Hague: Martinus Nijhoff.

Christy, M. (1981, June 2). "The Many Shades of du Plessix Gray." *The Boston Globe*.

Cope, J. F. (1973). *The Theatre and the Dream: From Metaphor to Form in Renaissance Drama*. Baltimore: Johns Hopkins UP.

Corbin, H. (1969). *Creative Imagination and the Sufism of Ibn 'Arabi*. Princeton: Princeton UP.

_____ (1972). "Mundus Imaginalis or the Imaginary and the Real." *Spring 1972*. Zürich: Spring Publications.

REFERENCES

———— (1977). *Spiritual Body and Celestial Earth: From Mazdean Iran to Shi 'ite Iran*. Trans. N. Pearson. Bollingen Series XCI:2. Princeton: Princeton UP.

———— (1980). *Avicenna and the Visionary Recital*. Irving, Texas: Spring Publications.

Croce, B. (1978). *Aesthetic; As Science of Expression and General Linguistic*. Boston: Nonpareil Books.

Daiches, D. (1960). *The Novel and the Modern World*. Chicago: University of Chicago Press.

Darwin, C. (1871). *The Descent of Man*. London: Murray.

Dillard, A. (1982). *Living by Fiction*. New York: Harper & Row.

Dodds, E. R. (1951). *The Greeks and the Irrational*. Berkeley: University of California Press.

Ekstein, R. (1965a). "Puppet Play of a Psychotic Adolescent Girl in the Psychotherapeutic Process." *The Psychoanalytic Study of the Child*, 20, 441-480.

———— (1965b). "The Working Alliance with the Monster." *Bulletin of the Menninger Clinic*, 4, 189-197.

Ellson, D. G. (1941). "Hallucinations Produced by Sensory Conditioning." *Journal of Experimental Psychology*, 78, 1-20.

Engell, J. (1981). *The Creative Imagination*. Cambridge: Harvard UP.

Erikson, E. (1950). *Childhood and Society*. New York: Norton.

Esquirol, J. E. D. (1833). "Sur les Illusions des Sens chez les Aliénee." *Archives Générales de Medicine*, Ser. 2, 1, 5-23.

———— (1838). *Des Maladies Mentales*. Paris: J. B. Bailliere.

Field, J. (1981). *A Life of One's Own*. Los Angeles: J. P. Tarcher.

Flavell, J. H. (1963). *The Developmental Psychology of Jean Piaget*. New York: D. Van Nostrand.

———— (1966). "Le Langage Privé." *Bulletin de Psychologie*, 19, 698-701.

Flavell, J. H., Higgins, J. B., and Klein, W. (1963). "Interview Study on the Speech of Self of a Sample of Faculty Children." Unpublished.

Franklin, M. (1981). "Play As the Creation of Imaginary Situations: The Role of Language." Eds. S. Wapner and B. Kaplan. *Toward a Holistic Developmental Psychology*. Hillsdale, New Jersey: Lawrence Erlbaum Associates.

Freeman, T., Cameron, J. L., and McGhie, A. (1966). *Studies on Psychosis*. New York. International UP.

Friedman, N. (1955). "Point of View in Fiction: The Development of a Critical Concept." *Publications of the MLA*, LXX, 1160-1184.

Freire, P. (1970). *Pedagogy of the Oppressed*. New York: Seabury.

Freire, P. and A. Faundez. (1989). *Learning to Question: A Pedagogy of Liberation*. New York: Continuum.

Freud, A., and Burlingham, D. (1942). *Infants Without Families*. New York: International UP.

Freud, S. (1957). *Formulations on the Two Principles of Mental Functioning. Standard Edition, XII*. London: Hogarth Press, 1911.

———— (1959). *Creative Writers and Day-Dreaming. Standard Edition, IX*. London: Hogarth Press, 1907.

———— (1963). *Introductory Lectures on Psychoanalysis. Standard Edition, XVI*. London: Hogarth Press, 1917.

———— (1964). *An Outline of Psycho-Analysis. Standard Edition, XXIII*. London: Hogarth Press, 1940.

———— (1965). *New Introductory Lectures on Psychoanalysis*. New York: Norton, 1932.

Fromm, E. (1976). *To Have or to Be*. New York: Harper & Row.

Gallagher, T., and Craig, H. (1978). "Structural Characteristics of Monologues in the Speech of Normal Children: Semantic and Conversational Aspects." *Journal of Speech and Hearing Research,* 21, 103-117.

Garvey, C. (1979). "Communicational Controls in Social Play." Ed. B. Sutton-Smith. *Play and Learning*. New York: Gardner Press.

Garvey C., and Berndt, R. (1977). "Organization of Pretend Play." *Catalogue of Selected Documents in Psychology,* 7, 107, Ms. 1589.

Gilligan, C. (1982). *In a Different Voice: Psychological Theory and Women's Development*. Cambridge: Harvard UP.

Gilson, E. (1957). *Painting and Reality*. Bollingen Series XXXV:4. New York: Pantheon Books.

Glick, J. (1981). *Piaget, Vygotsky, Werner*. First Biennial Conference, Developmental Psychology for the 1980's: Werner's Influences on Theory and Praxis. Clark University.

Goffman, E. (1981). *Forms of Talk*. Philadelphia: University of Pennsylvania Press.

Golomb, C. (1979). "Pretense Play: A Cognitive Perspective." Eds. N. S. Smith and M. Franklin. *Symbolic Functioning in Childhood*. Hillsdale, New Jersey: Lawrence Erlbaum Associates.

Gorky, M. (1920). *Reminiscences of Leo Nikolaevich Tolstoy*. Trans. S. S. Koteliansky and L. Woolf. New York: B. W. Huebsch.

Green, H. (1964). *I Never Promised You a Rose Garden*. New York: New American Library.

Greenson, R. R. (1954) "The Struggle Against Identification." *Journal of the American Psychoanalytic Association,* 2, 200-217.

Grotowski, J. (1968). *Towards a Poor Theatre*. New York: Simon & Schuster.

Griffiths, R. (1935). *A Study of Imagination in Early Childhood*. Westport, Conn.: Greenwood Press.

Gruhle, H. W. (1929)." Psycholgie des Abnormen." Ed. G. Aschaffenburg. *Handbuch der Vergleichende Psychologie*. Berlin: Springer.

REFERENCES

Gurney, E., and Myers, F. W. H. (1884). "A Theory of Apparitions." *Proceedings of the Society for Psychical Research*, 2, 109-136.

Halliday, M. A. (1964). *Explorations in the Functions of Language*. London: Arnold.

Harding, D. W. (1962). "Psychological Processes in the Reading of Fiction." *British Journal of Aesthetics*, II(2), 134-147.

Harriman, P. L. (1937). "Some Imaginary Companions of Older Subjects." *American Journal of Orthopsytchiatry*, 7, 368-370.

Hartmann, H. (1958). *Egopsychology and the Problem of Adaptation*. New York: International UP. 1939.

Harvey, W. J. (1965). *Character and the Novel*. Ithaca: Cornell UP.

Havens, L. (1962). "The Placement and Movement of Hallucinations in Space: Phenomenology and Theory." *International Journal of Psycho-Analysis*, 43(4), 426-435.

_____ (1981). Remarks at "Who Knows Best: Therapist or Patient?" Continuing Education Symposium, Massachusetts Mental Health Center.

Hermann, C. (1981). "The Virile System." Eds. E. Marks and I. de Courtivron. *New French Feminisms*. New York: Schocken Books.

Herron, R. E., and Sutton-Smith, B., eds. (1971). *Child's Play*. New York: Wiley.

Hilgard, E. R. (1973). "Dissociation Revisited." Eds. M. Henle, J. Jaynes, and J. J. Sullivan. *Historical Conceptions of Psychology*. New York: Springer.

Hillman, J. (1971). "Psychology: Monotheistic or Polytheistic?" *Spring 1971*. New York: Spring Publications.

_____ (1972). *The Myth of Analysis*. Evanston: Northwestem UP.

_____ (1973). "Abandoning the Child." *Eranos Jahrbuch 40*, 357-407. Leiden: Brill.

_____ (1975a). "Plotino, Ficino, and Vico as Precursors of Archetypal Psychology." *Loose Ends*. Zürich: Spring Publications.

_____ (1975b). *Re-Visioning Psychology*. New York: Harper & Row.

_____ (1977). "Psychotherapy's Inferiority Complex." *Eranos Jahrbuch 46*, 121-174. Leiden: Brill.

_____ (1982). "Anima Mundi: The Return of the Soul to the World." *Spring 1982*. Dallas: Spring Publications.

Horowitz, M. J. (1970). *Image Formation and Cognition*. New York: Appleton-Century-Crofts.

Horton, M. and P. Friere (1990). *We Make the Road by Walking: Conversations on Education and Social Change*. Philadelphia: Temple UP.

Howell, J. (1977). "Imaginary Companions: A Developmental Analysis." Unpublished.

Isaacs, S. (1933). *Social Development in Young Children*. London: Routledge & Sons.

_____ (1945). *Intellectual Growth in the Young Child.* London: Routledge & Sons.

James, H. (1934). *The Art of the Novel.* New York: Charles Scribner's Sons.

James W. (1892). *Psychology: A Briefer Course.* New York: Henry Holt.

Jaynes, J. (1976). *The Origin of Consciousness in the Breakdown of the Bicameral Mind.* Boston: Houghton, Mifflin.

Jung, C. G. (1936). "Fundamental Psychological Conceptions: A Report of Five Lectures by Jung." London Lectures, London Multigraph Typescript, 214-235. Later published as "The Tavistock Lectures." *Collected Works of C. G. Jung.* Vol. 18.

_____ (1937). *Psychological Analysis of Nietzsche's Zarathustra.* Privately mimeographed seminar notes, prepared by Mary Foote.

_____ (1954). "The Practice of Psychotherapy." Trans. R. F. C. Hull. *Collected Works of C. G. Jung.* Vol. 16. Bollingen Series XX. Princeton: Princeton UP.

_____ (1961). *Memories, Dreams, Reflections.* Ed. A. Jaffé. Trans. Richard and Clara Winston. New York: Alfred Knopf.

_____ (1968a). "Alchemical Studies." Trans. R. F. C. Hull. *Collected Works of C. G. Jung.* Vol. 13. Bollingen Series XX. Princeton: Princeton UP.

_____ (1968b). *Analytical Psychology: Its Theory and Practice.* New York: Vintage.

_____ (1968c). "The Archetypes and the Collective Unconscious." Trans. R. F. C. Hull. *Collected Works of C. G. Jung,* Vol. 9 (Part I). Bollingen Series XX. Princeton: Princeton UP.

_____ (1969). "The Structure and Dynamics of the Psyche." Trans. R. F. C. Hull. *Collected Works of C. G. Jung.* Vol. 8. Bollingen Series XX. Princeton: Princeton UP.

_____ (1971). "Psychological Types." Trans. R. F. C. Hull. *Collected Works of C. G. Jung,* Vol. 6. Bollingen Series XX. Princeton: Princeton UP.

_____ (1973). *Selected Letters of C. G. Jung.* Eds. G. Adler and A. Jaffé. Princeton: Princeton UP.

Jung, C. G. and Kerényi, C. (1949). *Essays On a Science of Mythology: The Myth of the Divine Child and the Mysteries of Eleusis.* Trans. R. F. C. Hull. Bollingen Series XX. Princeton: Princeton UP.

Kaplan, B. (1959). "The Study of Language in Psychiatry." Ed. S. Arieti. *American Handbook of Psychiatry.* Vol. 3. New York: Basic Books.

_____ (1960). "Lectures on Developmental Psychology." Papers presented at Worcester State Hospital and Clark University (Revised in 1980).

_____ (1974). "Strife of Systems: Tension Between Organismic and Developmental Points of View." Heinz Werner Lecture, Clark University, Worcester.

_____ (1981a). "Basking in Burke." Clark University, Worcester.

REFERENCES

_____ (1981b). "The Development of Language in Relation to Mental Health." Paper presented at colloquia on The Development of Language and Its Relation to Mental Health, Cornell University Medical College, New York City.

_____ (1981c). "Psychology as a Science." Paper presented at Meetings of the Massachusetts Psychological Association, Clark University, Worcester.

_____ (1981d). "Radical Metaphor, Aesthetic and the Origin of Language." (Original version appeared in *Review of Existential Psychology and Psychiatry*, 1962.)

_____ (1983a). "A Trio of Trials." Ed. R. M. Lerner. *Developmental Psychology: Historical and Philosophical Perspectives*. Hillsdale, New Jersey: Lawrence Erlbaum Associates.

_____ (1983b). "Genetic Dramatism: Old Wine in New Bottles." Eds. S. Wapner and B. Kaplan. *Toward a Holistic Developmental Psychology*. Hillsdale, New Jersey: Lawrence Erlbaum Associates.

Kaplan, B., and Crockett, W. H. (1968). "Developmental Modes of Analysis." Eds. E. Aronson and R. P. Abelson. *Theories of Cognitive Consistency: A Sourcebook*. Chicago: Rand McNally.

Kaplan, E. (1952). "An Experimental Study on Inner Speech as Contrasted with External Speech." Unpublished doctoral dissertation, Clark University.

Kernberg, O. (1980). *Internal World and External Reality*. New York: Aronson.

Kiely, R. (1980). *Beyond Egotism: The Fiction of James Joyce, Virginia Woolf and D. H. Lawrence*. Cambridge: Harvard UP.

Kierkegaard, S. (1941). *The Sickness Unto Death*. Princeton: Princeton UP.

Klein, M. (1975a). *Envy and Gratitude*. Boston: Delacorte Press.

_____ (1915b). *The Psychoanalysis of Children*. Boston: Delacorte Press.

Klein, W. L. (1963). "An Investigation of the Spontaneous Speech of Children During Problem Solving." Unpublished doctoral dissertation, University of Rochester.

Kohlberg, L., Yaeger, J., and Hjertholm, E. (1968). "Private Speech: Four Studies and a Review of Theories." *Child Development*, 39, 691-735.

Krohn, A. and Mayman, M. (1974). "Object Representation in Dreams and Projective Tests." *Bulletin of the Menninger Clinic*, 38, 445-466.

Landor, W. S. (1915). *Imaginary Conversations*. London: Oxford UP.

Lawrence, D. H. (1962). *Collected Letters of D. H. Lawrence*. Vol. 1. Ed. H. T. Moore. New York: Viking Press.

Leuret, F. (1834). *Fragments Psychologiques sur la Folie*. Paris: Crochard.

Lewinsohn, P. M. (1968). "Characteristics of Patients with Hallucinations." *Journal of Clinical Psychology*, 24, 423.

Lockhart, R. A. (1975). "Mary's Dog is an Ear Mother: Listening to the Voices of Psychosis." *Psychological Perspectives*, 6, 144-160.

Lovejoy, A. O. (1961). *The Reason, the Understanding and Time.* Baltimore: Johns Hopkins UP.

Lowe, M. (1975). "Trends in the Development of Representational Play in Infants from One to Three Years—An Observational Study." *Journal of Child Psychology and Psychiatry,* 16, 33-47.

MacMurray, J. (1957). "The Self as Agent." *The Form of the Personal.* New York: Harper & Row.

Maritain, J. (1953). *Creative Intuition in Art and Poetry.* Bollingen Series XXXV:I. New York: Pantheon Books.

Mead, G. H. (1924-1925). "The Genesis of the Self and Social Control." *International Journal of Ethics,* 35, 251-277.

_____ (1934). *Mind, Self and Society.* Chicago: University of Chicago Press.

_____ (1936). *Movements of Thought in the Nineteenth Century.* Chicago: University of Chicago Press.

_____ (1978). "The Social Self." *Psychiatry,* 41, 178-183.

Meichenbaum, D. (1977). *Cognitive-Behavior Modification: An Integrative Approach.* New York; Plenum Press.

Meichenbaum, D., & Goodman, S. (1979). "Clinical Use of Private Speech and Critical Questions about Its Study in Natural Settings." Ed. G. Zivin. *The Development of Self-Regulation through Private Speech.* New York: Wiley.

Meissner, W. W. (1981). *Internalization in Psychoanalysis.* New York: Inter. UP.

Merleau-Ponty, M. (1962). *The Phenomenology of Perception.* London: Routledge & Kegan Paul.

_____ (1973). *The Prose of the World.* Evanston: Northwestern UP.

Michea, C. F. (1846). *Du Délire des Sensations.* Paris: Label.

Miller, A. (1981). *The Drama of the Gifted Child.* New York: Basic Books.

Miller, D. L. (1974). *The New Polytheism.* New York: Harper & Row.

Miller, D. (1973). *George Herbert Mead: Self, Language and World.* Chicago: University of Chicago Press.

Miller, H. (1939). *Henry Miller on Writing.* New York: New Directions.

Milosz, C. (1974). *Bells in Winter.* New York: Ecco Press.

Moore, S. (1974). *The Stanislavski System.* New York: Viking Press.

Moreau (de Tours), J. (1845). *Du Hachisch et de l'Aliénation Mentale.* Paris: Mason.

Morris, W., ed.. (1969). *The American Heritage Dictionary of the English Language.* New York: American Heritage/Houghton Mifflin.

Morrisette, B. (1961-1962). "The New Novel in France." *Chicago Review,* 15(3).

Muchnic, H. (1980, October 12). "Chosen and Used by Art." *The New York Times Book Review.*

Nicolich, L. (1977). "Beyond Sensorimotor Intelligence: Assessment of Symbolic Maturity through Analysis of Pretend Play." *Merrill-Palmer Quarterly*, 23, 89-99.

Niebuhr, R. (1955). *The Self and the Dramas of History*. New York: Scribner's.

Ochs, E., and Schiefflin, eds. (1979). *Developmental Pragmatics*. New York: Academic Press.

O'Connor, F. (1961). *Mystery and Manners*. New York: Farrar, Straus & Giroux.

Olson, E. (1942). "Sailing to Byzantium: Prolegomena to a Poetics of the Lyric." *The University of Kansas City Review*, 8, 3.

O'Neill, E. (1981). "An Interview with Eugene O'Neill." WGBH Radio, Boston.

Otto, W. F. (1981). *Dionysos: Myth and Cult*. Dallas: Spring Publications.

Oxford English Dictionary (longer). (1933). Oxford: Clarendon Press.

Oxford English Dictionary (shorter). (1933). Oxford: Clarendon Press.

Parish, E. (1897). *Hallucinations and Illusions: A Study of the Fallacies of Perception*. New York: Charles Scribner's Sons.

Peller, L. E. (1954). "Libidinal Phases, Ego Development, and Play." *The Psychoanalytic Study of the Child*, 9, 178-198.

Perky, C. W. (1910). "An Experimental Study of Imagination." *American Journal of Psychology*, 21, 422-452.

Pfuetze, P. (1973). *Self, Society, Existence: Human Nature and Dialogue in the Thought of George Herbert Mead and Martin Buber*. Westport, Conn.: Greenwood Press.

Piaget, J. (1955). *The Language and Thought of the Child*. New York: New American Library.

_____ (1960). *The Child's Conception of the World*. Totowa, New Jersey: Littlefield, Adams.

_____ (1962a). *Comments on Vygotsky's Critical Remarks Concerning "The Language and Thought of the Child," and "Judgment and Reasoning in the Child."* Cambridge: MIT Press.

_____ (1962b). *Play, Dreams and Imitation*. New York: Norton.

_____ (1971). "Response to Brian Sutton-Smith." Eds. R. E. Herron and B. Sutton-Smith. *Child's Play*. New York: Wiley.

Pines, M. (1978, September). "Invisible Playmates." *Psychology Today*, 38-42.

Pirandello, L. (1952). *Naked Masks: Five Plays by Pirandello*. Ed. E. Bentley. New York: Dutton.

Plato. (1961). *The Collected Dialogues*. Eds. E. Hamilton and H. Cairns. Bollingen Series LXXI. Princeton: Princeton UP.

Radin, P. (1954). *Monotheism Among Primitive Peoples*. (Ethnographical Museum). Basel: Bollingen Foundations, Special Publication 4.

Rambert, M. L. (1949). *Children in Conflict: Twelve Years of Psychoanalytic Practice.* New York: International UP.

Repina, T. A. (1971). "Development of Imagination." Eds. A. Zaporozhets and D. B. Elkonin. *Psychology of Preschool Children.* Cambridge: MIT Press.

Robinson, M. (1980). *Housekeeping.* New York: Bantam Books.

Rogers, R. (1970). *The Double in Literature.* Detroit: Wayne State UP.

Rubin, K. (1979). "The Impact of the Natural Setting on Private Speech." Ed. G. Zivin. *The Development of Self-Regulation through Private Speech.* New York: Wiley.

Rycroft, C. (1979). *The Innocence of Dreams.* New York: Pantheon Books.

Sach, J. (1980). "The Role of Adult-Child Play in Language Development." Ed. K. H. Rubin. *New Directions for Child Development.* Vol 9.

Sampson, E. (1993). "Identity Politics: Challenges to Psychology's Understanding." *American Psychologist, 48,* 12, 1219-1230.

Sanders, T. G. (1976). *The Spirit Possession of Alejandro Mamani.* Hanover, New Hampshire: Wheelock Educational Resources.

Sarbin, T. (1967). "The Concept of Hallucination." *Journal of Personality,* 35(3), 359-380.

Sarbin, T., and Juhasz, J. (1967). "The Historical Background of the Concept of Hallucinations." *Journal of the History of the Behavioral Sciences,* 3, 339-358.

Sartre, J. P. (1949). *What is Literature?* New York: Philosophical Library.

Schafer, R. (1968). *Aspects of Internalization.* New York: International UP.

_____ (1970). "The Psychoanalytic Vision of Reality." *International Journal of Psycho-Analysis,* 51 (3), 279-297.

_____ (1976). *A New Language for Psychoanalysis.* New Haven: Yale UP.

Schimek, J. (1975). "A Critical Re-Examination of Freud's Concept of Unconscious Representation." *International Journal of Psycho-Analysis,* 2, 171-187.

Scholes, R. E., and Kellogg, R. (1966). *The Nature of Narrative.* New York: Oxford UP.

Schreiber, F. R. (1973). *Sybil.* New York: Warner.

Schumaker, W. (1960). *Literature and the Irrational: A Study in Anthropological Backgrounds.* Englewood Cliffs, New Jersey: Prentice-Hall.

Searles, H. (1960). *Collected Papers on Schizophrenia and Related Subjects.* New York: International UP.

Sechehaye, M. (1951). *The Autobiography of a Schizophrenic Girl.* New York: Grune & Stratton.

Selman, R. and L. Schultz (1990). *Making a Friend in Youth.* Chicago: University of Chicago Press.

Shields, M. M. (1978). "Some Communication Skills of Young Children: A Study of Dialogue in the Nursery Schools." Eds. R. C. Campbell and P. T. Smith. *Recent Advances in the Psychology of Language.* New York: Plenum.

_____ (1979). "Monologue, Dialogue and Egocentric Speech by Children in Nursery Schools." Eds. O. K. Garnica and M. L. King. *Language, Children and Society*. New York: Pergamon Press.

Sidgewick, H., et al. (1894). "Report on the Census of Hallucinations." *Proceedings of the Society for Psychical Research*, 34, 25-394.

Singer, J. (1973). *The Child's World of Make Believe: Experimental Studies of Imaginative Play*. New York: Academic Press.

Slama-Cazacu, T. (1976). *Dialogue in Children*. The Hague: Mouton.

Smith, H. (1976). *Forgotten Truth*. New York: Harper & Row.

Sperling, O. (1954). "An Imaginary Companion Representing a Presage of the Superego." *The Psychoanalytic Study of the Child*, 9, 252-258.

Stanislavski, S. (1936). *An Actor Prepares*. New York: Theatre Arts Books.

_____ (1948). *My Life in Art*. New York: Theatre Arts Books.

Stevens, W. (1978). *The Collected Poems of Wallace Stevens*. New York: Alfred Knopf.

Stoney, B. (1974). *Enid Blyton: A Biography*. London: Hodder.

Straus, E. W. (1958). "Aesthesiology and Hallucinations." Eds. R. May, E. Angel, and H. F. Ellenberger. *Existence*. New York: Basic Books.

_____ (1966). *Phenomenological Psychology*. New York: Basic Books.

Strong, A. L. (1909). *The Psychology of Prayer*. Chicago: University of Chicago Press.

Sukenick, R. (1967). *Wallace Stevens: Musing the Obscure*. New York: New York UP.

Sutton-Smith, B. (1971). "Piaget on Play: A Critique." Eds. R. E. Herron and B. Sutton-Smith. *Child's Play*. New York: Wiley.

Szanto, G. H. (1972). *Narrative Consciousness*. Austin: University of Texas Press.

Thomas, L. (1974). *The Medusa and the Snail*. New York: Viking Press.

Toulmin, S. (1981). "Epistemology and Developmental Psychology." Ed. E. S. Gollin. *Developmental Plasticity*. New York: Academic Press.

Trollope, A. (1930). *Trollope: An Autobiography*. Edinburgh: William Blackwood & Sons, 1833.

Tuveson, E. L. (1974). *Imagination as a Means of Grace*. New York: Gordian Press.

Van den Berg, J. H. (1982a). "On Hallucinating: Critical Historical Overview and Guidelines for Further Study." Eds. A. J. de Koning and F. A. Jenner. *Phenomenology and Psychiatry*. New York: Grune & Stratton.

_____ (1982b). "The Schizophrenic Patient: Anthropological Considerations." Eds. A. J. de Koning and F. A. Jenner. *Phenomenology and Psychiatry*. New York: Grune & Stratton.

Verene, D. P. (1979). "Categories and the Imagination." Eds. R. Staley and D. Pariser. *Aesthetics and Culture, Presentations on Art Education and Research*, 5.

Vygotsky, L. S. (1962). *Thought and Language*. Cambridge: MIT Press.

_____(1978). "The Role of Play in Development." *Mind in Society: The development of Higher Psychological Processes.* Cambridge: Harvard UP.

Walker, A. (1983). *In Search of Our Mothers' Gardens.* New York: Harcourt Brace Jovanovich.

Warneck, M. (1909). *Die Religion der Batak.* Leipzig: T. Weicher.

Watkins, M. (1974). "The Waking Dream in European Psychotherapy." *Spring 1974.* Zürich: Spring Publications.

_____ (1978). "Self and Object Representation in the Dreams of Schizophrenics and Non-schizophrenics." Unpublished Master's Thesis, Clark University.

_____ (1981a, July). "The Development of Imaginal Dialogues in Psychotherapy: Case Examples." Lecture at Wright Institute, Berkeley.

_____ (1981b). "Six Approaches to the Image in Art Therapy." *Spring 1981.* Dallas: Spring Publications.

_____ (1984). *Waking Dreams.* Dallas: Spring Publications. (1976).

Watson, M., and Fischer, K. W. (1977). "A Developmental Sequence of Agent Use in Late Infancy." *Child Development,* 48, 828-836.

Webster's New Collegiate Dictionary. (1960). Springfield, Mass.: Merriam.

Weir, R. H. (1962). *Language in the Crib.* The Hague: Mouton.

Wemer, H. (1948). *Comparative Psychology of Mental Development.* New York: International UP.

Werner, H., and Kaplan, B. (1984). *Symbol Formation.* Hillsdale, New Jersey: Lawrence Erlbaum Associates (1963).

Whitehead, A. N. (1925). *Science and the Modern World.* New York: New American Library.

Whitman, W. (1959). *Leaves of Grass.* New York: Viking Press.

Winnicott, D. W. (1971). *Playing and Reality.* New York: International UP.

Woolf, V. (1929). *A Room of One's Own.* New York: Harcourt, Brace & World.

_____ (1953). *The Common Reader.* New York: Harcourt, Brace & World (Originally published, 1925).

Zivin, G., ed. (1979). *The Development of Self-Regulation through Private Speech.* New York: Wiley.

Zucker, K. (1928). "Experimentelles über Sinnestäuschungen." *Archiv der Psychiatrischen Neurologie,* 83, 706-754.

ABOUT THE AUTHOR

MARY WATKINS is a clinical and developmental psychologist and one of the original members of the group of psychotherapists, writers, and psychologists who founded Archetypal Psychology in the 1970s. A core faculty member and the Coordinator of Community and Ecological Fieldwork and Research in the Depth Psychology M.A./Ph.D. Program at Pacifica Graduate Institute, Watkins has written numerous essays on the confluence of liberation psychology and depth psychology and is the author of *Waking Dreams, Invisible Guests: The Development of Imaginal Dialogues,* and the co-author of *Talking With Young Children About Adoption.*